Data Safety Monitoring Boards

Basic Bioethics

Arthur Caplan, editor

A complete list of the books in the Basic Bioethics series appears at the back of this book.

Data Safety Monitoring Boards

A Bioethical Perspective

Deborah R. Barnbaum

foreword by Janet Wittes

The MIT Press
Cambridge, Massachusetts
London, England

The MIT Press
Massachusetts Institute of Technology
77 Massachusetts Avenue, Cambridge, MA 02139
mitpress.mit.edu

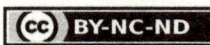
The MIT Press would like to thank the anonymous peer reviewers who provided
comments on drafts of this book. The generous work of academic experts is essential
for establishing the authority and quality of our publications. We acknowledge with
gratitude the contributions of these otherwise uncredited readers.

This book was set in Stone Serif and Stone Sans by Westchester Publishing Services.
Printed and bound in the United States of America.

Library of Congress Cataloging-in-Publication Data

Names: Barnbaum, Deborah R., 1967- author.
Title: Data safety monitoring boards : a bioethical perspective / Deborah
    Barnbaum.
Description: Cambridge : The MIT Press, 2025. | Series: Basic bioethics |
    Includes bibliographical references and index.
Identifiers: LCCN 2024039690 (print) | LCCN 2024039691 (ebook) |
    ISBN 9780262552745 (paperback) | ISBN 9780262383622 (epub) |
    ISBN 9780262383639 (pdf)
Subjects: LCSH: Data safety monitoring boards (Medicine) | Clinical
    trials—Evaluation. | Medical ethics.
Classification: LCC R852.55 .B37 2025 (print) | LCC R852.55 (ebook) |
    DDC 174.2—dc23/eng/20250411
LC record available at https://lccn.loc.gov/2024039690
LC ebook record available at https://lccn.loc.gov/2024039691

10 9 8 7 6 5 4 3 2 1

EU Authorised Representative: Easy Access System Europe, Mustamäe tee 50, 10621
Tallinn, Estonia | Email: gpsr.requests@easproject.com

Dedicated to those brave enough to help others by serving in research. Thank you.

Contents

Foreword

Janet Wittes

We biostatisticians consider data safety monitoring boards (DSMBs) to rest firmly in our bailiwick. Evidence for the centrality of our ownership abounds. As Deborah Barnbaum describes in her compelling monograph, when the National Heart, Lung, and Blood Institute (NHLBI) sought guidance on how to monitor ongoing data from randomized controlled trials, they established a committee to provide advice to the institute. As the head of that committee, they chose Professor Bernard Greenberg, the chair of the Biostatistics Department at the University of North Carolina, Chapel Hill. The report, produced in 1967 and widely available soon thereafter, has influenced controlled clinical trials ever since. Writing about DSMBs and developing technical approaches to data monitoring has become somewhat of a cottage industry for biostatisticians. The authors of textbooks and many papers about the topic have been biostatisticians. Charters of DSMBs usually contain a paragraph specifying that the quorum needed for meetings must include the chair of the committee and a biostatistician member. An essential part of graduate school courses in clinical trials includes statistical methodology of data monitoring. Senior faculty often encourage their postdoctoral biostatistics students to seize the opportunity to sit on a DSMB when offered the chance, or to attend meetings as a "trainee."

My own experience with DSMBs dates from 1983 when I became the branch chief of the Biostatistics Research Branch at NHBLI. I was already familiar with institutional review boards, which Barnbaum in chapter 1 clearly differentiates from DSMBs. Very early in my tenure at NHLBI (in my memory it was on day 1, but I suspect my memory is faulty), two members of the branch—Gordon Lan and Kent Bailey—gave me emphatic advice. "You," they said, "as chief, are allowed to attend as many DMSB meetings as you want." *Go to them all*, they urged. They emphasized that by listening to the discussion, I would gain invaluable understanding of many aspects of randomized controlled trials as well as important insights into how physicians think about their patients and about data. I gladly heeded their advice. During my seven years at the branch, I attended as many DSMB meetings as possible. The trials varied in length, in the severity of the diseases they were studying, in the populations participating in them, and in the clinical outcomes they were assessing. I could not have had a better education. After leaving the branch in 1990, I spent the next thirty years running a small statistical consulting company that served as the independent statistical reporting group (ISRG) for many industry-run randomized trials. In those three decades, I sat as a member of three types of groups associated with DSMBs. First, for the National Institute of Health, the Veteran's Administration, the World Health Organization, and industry, I sat on, and sometimes chaired, DSMBs (more commonly called data monitoring committees in industry). Second, I led the ISRG for many trials sponsored by industry. And finally, for some industry-sponsored trials, I served as a member of the executive committee of randomized controlled trials and was thus the recipient of the recommendation letters from the DSMB.

I learned a tremendous amount from other members of DSMBs. Most importantly, I observed how different disciplines think about interpreting emerging data. All these DSMBs included physicians and at least one biostatistician. A few also included an "ethicist," either a person with formal training in bioethics or someone assigned the role of the "ethicist." What has struck me in my experience, and is emphasized in this book, is what people formally trained in biomedical ethics contribute. They bring a rigor grounded in philosophy; it is from those that I have learned the most. Much of what they taught me has dealt with the informed consent form— the document discussed with the investigator and signed when a potential participant is about to join a trial. In some trials, new information emerges that leads to further discussion between the investigator and the participant about benefits and risks. A revised informed consent form is the means by which, during the course of a trial, participants receive a document describing the updated information. The important role of bioethicists in writing and reviewing informed consent forms is the topic of chapter 2.

The first case that uprooted my prior understanding of the distinction between ethicists with formal training in philosophy and those without occurred when I was chairing the National Eye Institute's (NEI) DSMC ("C" for "committee" in NEI-speak) for the Age-Related Eye Disease study (AREDS) (Age-Related Eye Disease Study Research Group 2001). AREDS was investigating whether daily supplementation with a cocktail of antioxidants, including beta-carotene, would delay the progression of age-related macular degeneration in high-risk adults aged fifty-five to eighty. Participants were randomized in a masked manner to the antioxidant cocktail or to placebo. (NEI-funded studies use the word "masked" instead of "blinded.") The study began recruitment in 1992, a time during which supplementation with antioxidants was popularly viewed as likely beneficial to health in general and to the eye in particular; antioxidants were certainly not considered likely to be harmful. Two years after AREDS started, the ATBC trial (Alpha-Tocopherol, Beta-Carotene Cancer Prevention Study Group 1994), a large-scale randomized controlled trial of male smokers in Finland, reported that compared to placebo, supplementation with the antioxidants vitamin E and beta-carotene appeared to lead to an increased rate of lung cancer and total mortality. Given how unexpected the findings were, and because the population in ATBC differed so dramatically from the population in AREDS, the DSMC did not consider the results necessarily relevant to AREDS. Nonetheless, the alarming nature of lung cancer and death led us to be cautious. We recommended that the NEI inform all AREDS participants about the findings from ATBC. Further, we asked the NEI to remind AREDS participants that they were free to stop or continue taking their masked study medication and to urge them to continue follow-up even if they stopped their medication. The recommendations were both unanimous and not difficult to make; as we expected, the NEI took our advice.

What was not difficult in 1994 became agonizing in 1996 when two studies appeared in the same issue of the *New England Journal of Medicine*. The CARET study, a double-blind randomized controlled trial comparing beta-carotene to placebo in men and women, showed that smokers randomized to beta-carotene experienced an increase in lung cancer incidence and total mortality relative to those randomized to placebo (Omenn et al. 1996). The Physicians Health Study, however, which compared beta-carotene to placebo in male physicians, showed no such increase in either the population as a whole or in smokers (Hennekens et al. 1996). We were now faced with a dilemma—AREDS, like the Physicians Health Study, was showing no evidence of harm, but we struggled with how to acknowledge the CARET results, which were disturbingly similar to the results in ATBC. We considered doing nothing—after all, the emerging data from AREDS showed no evidence of harm. Or we could recommend stopping the trial entirely But that seemed like an overreaction. Then the late Robert Veatch, our ethicist, spoke up. Now I confess that prior to the reports from ATBC and CARET, I had sometimes found ethicists to be irritating members of DSMBs. During meetings, some seemed to act as if they considered themselves, but not the rest of us, "ethical." In retrospect, I was unfair. Nonetheless, whatever I had thought prior to 1996, my view changed dramatically the day Professor Veatch walked us through how to think about making a recommendation in light of ATBC, CARET, and the Physicians Health Study. He led us through a principled, technical, philosophically based set of possible choices, focusing on the science learned through the three studies, as well as the emerging data from AREDS. He emphasized the difference between results in smokers and nonsmokers, in men and women. He stressed the importance of informing the participants in AREDS about the results of all three other trials. Under his guidance, we formulated a recommendation, which the NEI implemented, that smokers in AREDS should seriously consider stopping any supplementation that contained beta-carotene or its placebo. I do not know what we would have concluded had Professor Veatch not been on the committee, but his sober, rational, compassionate thinking led us to a recommendation with which we were all comfortable. For further information about how these recommendations played out, see AREDS report no. 1 (The Age-Related Eye Disease Study Group, 1999).

At the same time that AREDS was recruiting and following patients, the Women's Health Initiative (WHI) (Wittes et al. 2007), a set of four interrelated trials in postmenopausal women, was in progress. Here again, I chaired the DSMB. While in AREDS our quandary stemmed from worrisome, but inconsistent, results emanating from trials outside our own, in the WHI the problem arose from data within the WHI itself. We were seeing that the rates of heart attacks, strokes, and pulmonary emboli were higher in women randomized to hormone therapy than in those randomized to placebo. Again, we were fortunate to have an extremely thoughtful bioethicist on the board, Professor LeRoy Walters. We were all strongly convinced that the NHLBI was obligated to inform the investigators of these observed increases and that they, in turn, were responsible for explaining to the participants what the data were showing because the ongoing data differed substantially from what the informed consent form had said. However, we did not want to recommend terminating the trial because we did not know whether the long-term use of hormone therapy would indeed prove beneficial. What Veatch had done for the AREDS DSMC, Walters did for the WHI DSMB—he demonstrated a formal approach to thinking about presenting ongoing data to participants in a way that fully informed them but that did not compromise the integrity of the trial.

Both the AREDS and the WHI monitoring committees faced the problem of updating information about risks to participants already enrolled in ongoing trials. Sometimes, the issues of informed consent are very complicated when investigators are initially recruiting potential participants. For example, I was a member of a DSMB charged with assessing safety and efficacy of an ongoing industry-sponsored trial, MERITAGE, that was testing the efficacy of targeted radiation for treatment of wet age-related macular degeneration (Petrarca et al. 2014). We, the DSMB, struggled with how the investigators should explain the risks of radiation to participants who were considering entering the trial. The late Professor Baruch Brody, the bioethicist on the DSMB, taught the rest of us to put ourselves in the head of a potential participant who did not necessarily understand what "radiation" meant (were they thinking of atomic bombs?) and to read the informed consent form as if we were such a person. Brody's intelligent, careful parsing of the language in the informed consent document provided me with tools to read such documents in the future. After my experience with these three trials, and the training I had received from these three bioethicists, I relied on informed consent documents to aid in my own understanding of trials and how to explain risks to potential participants in those trials.

As a final example, consider the NEI-sponsored CALEC trial (Jurkunas, Johns, and Armant 2022), which Barnbaum discusses in chapter 3. We were lucky that Barnbaum was our bioethicist because, as she explains in the book, the risks involved in participation were very different from risks in usual trials. At each of our meetings, she brought insights to the rest of the committee that reflected her special expertise. I will not write more about CALEC here—chapter 3 carefully presents the unique aspects of risks in that trial. The chapter proceeds with an insightful discussion of how bioethicists think about the balance of benefits and risk.

Prior to reading this book, I felt lucky that in the four situations described above, where the DSMB was faced with issues of how to describe the trial to participants, we had a formally trained ethicist on the committee. They helped us formulate how best to describe risks to potential participants (MERITAGE and CALEC) and how to react to emerging evidence of harms (AREDS and the WHI). This book has made me laugh at myself because I now realize this was not luck; each of these DSMBs had a technically trained bioethicist as a member because the sponsors (NEI, NHLBI, and the device company NeoVista) had understood the importance of the role of such a person. Looking back on DSMBs that faced difficult problems, but which did not have a bioethicist on the board, I wonder now how we would have proceeded if we in fact had a bioethicist as a member. My experience with bioethicists has taught me to rely on the informed consent form to parse out what participants had been told before they joined the trial, but I can think of trials where we, the DSMB, struggled with what recommenda-tion would ensure protection of the rights of participants. I strongly suspect we would have been better served had a bioethicist been a member.

Just as I find myself realizing that having a bioethicist on the committees that I discussed was not a matter of luck, I am amused, and grateful, for how much I have learned from this book. A confession: I did not understand the difference between a "bioethicist" and a "patient advocate"—in chapter 2, Barnbaum explains the difference between the two roles in a way that is crystal clear. Also, before reading this book, I was unable to grasp what *equipoise* means. I assumed my failure to understand the word reflected a lack of knowledge of the basics of clinical trials, a field in which I have worked for nearly half a century. Chapter 4, which presents a host of definitions of *equipoise*, was a revelation. Knowing that bioethicists themselves differ about the meaning of *equipoise* came as a relief. In the chapter, Barnbaum makes the very valuable point that whether a study is in equipoise depends on who is making the judgment—researchers, the clinical community, or participants.

Recruitment, retention, and adherence are topics well known to clinical trialists. Often investigators focus on recruitment but spend too little effort on enhancing retention to the trial and adherence to the protocol. How these aspects relate to bioethics is the subject of chapter 5.

The first five chapters are accessible to those of us who are not con-versant with the philosophical background familiar to bioethicists. The last chapter, which is much more technical, provides important insights. The "consequentialist ethic" Barnbaum describes was new to me. I suspect clinicians and other statisticians who have been involved in DSMBs for years will, like me, find the discussion of theories of ethics illuminating.

As I read the book and thought about the lessons I learned, I found myself mulling over two overarching questions: When does a DSMB need a bioethicist as a member? And what are the distinctions between biostatisticians and bioethicists with respect to DSMBs? The facile answer to the first question is "Every DSMB should have a bioethicist," but that is not realistic. There are too few bioethicists to fill all these slots, and most trials probably do not involve questions of a serious ethical nature. To answer, "A trial that might raise ethical problems should have an ethicist on the DSMB," is of little help—one never knows a priori how likely an ethical issue is to arise. So maybe the answer is the one we biostatisticians use so often: "It depends." Certainly, one can argue that a bioethicist is necessary for trials that proceed with a waiver of consent. Other trials that appear to need a bioethicist are those studying a population that is especially vulnerable, assessing an outcome that has serious health consequences, or investigating a truly novel or risky intervention. Members of DSMBs that do not include a bioethicist should have the right, even the obligation, to request advice from a bioethicist experienced in clinical trials if the trial is facing an ethical dilemma. As the community of trialists, including bioethicists, gains more experience with bioethicists on DSMBs, we shall collectively learn when they are needed, when they are useful but not necessary, and when their presence is unlikely to be helpful. This book's discussion of ethics in trial monitoring is a positive step toward educating the community of trialists.

Finally, a few words about the question of the difference between bioethicists and biostatisticians with respect to our role on DSMBs. In some ways, we are both interlopers. After all, it is the physicians who treat; the results of a trial may affect how they deal with their future patients. Bioethicists and biostatisticians do not treat patients; we help clinicians design, analyze, and interpret the trials in a way that enhances the ability of the trials to answer questions that will best serve patients. We biostatisticians look at the data, weigh benefit and risk quantitatively—as best we can—and ask ourselves what the data are saying. Our role is to explain to the others on the committee the statistical methodology being used and the inferences that can reliably be drawn from the ongoing data. Sponsors see us as essential to the process of data monitoring, partly because so many regulatory decisions require unbiased statistical analysis. Other members of the DSMB defer to us. The word *statistics* scares some other members of the DSMB. They will make statements like, "Statistics was my worst course in college," or "Will the statisticians tell me if this could have occurred by chance?" Our expertise is recognized; the other members do not think they can take our place. It is our responsibility to explain what we are doing in a jargon-free way that allows the other members to be intelligently engaged in discussion.

The story is different for bioethicists. They also look at the data; but they ask if the data are consistent with what participants have been told about potential risks and benefits. The word *ethics*, in contrast to *statistics*, is part of our daily vernacular—we all think we know what is "ethical," and we consider ourselves to be "ethical" or, at the very least, not unethical. Thus, bioethicists face a hurdle that we biostatisticians do not need to jump over. As we all sit around the DSMB table, the physicians tell us about the biology of the intervention and the progress of the disease. The rest of us listen and learn; we know they have expertise the rest of us do not have. We biostatisticians interpret data and explain the statistical methodology being used. The others do not think they have the expertise to do our job. But bioethicists have a problem. Throughout the book, Barnbaum, either explicitly or implicitly, emphasizes that *ethics* in common parlance differs from *ethics* in the technical sense. Ethicist members of a DSMB must remember that the rest of us may not appreciate that distinction, and therefore, they must recognize the important role they have in teaching the rest of the committee about the formal structure that informs their thinking.

This book promises to enrich the DSMB ecosystem. It should encourage the community of clinical trialists to embrace inclusion of technically trained ethicists on DSMBs. I hope that many bioethicists, on reading this book, will want to join the community of those involved in DSMBs. When they do, they should use as their template the kind of thinking that Barnbaum so eloquently describes.

Acknowledgements

Expressing gratitude is a lot like an informed consent: Neither are "one-and-done," and there's always the fear that something, or someone, important has been left out.

If intrinsic value is measured by the number of persons for whom good is promoted, and the amount of good promoted for each person, then nothing I've done in the last decade has greater value than my membership on numerous DSMBs. It has been an honor to work with each, and each has taught me something new. My longest-standing membership on a monitoring committee has been with the DRCRnet (formerly the Diabetic Retinopathy Clinical Research Network). I've learned more than can be measured from current and past members, including Stephen Wisniewski (current chair), John Connett (past chair), Lee M. Jampol, Harry E. Flynn, Gary W. Abrams, Ruth S. Weinstock, Paul Sternberg, Kyle Rudser, and the late Saul Genuth. Thank you for all you've shared. I'm similarly indebted to Roy Beck, Adam Glassman, and the rest of the team at the Jaeb Center for Health Research.

My contacts at the NIH are among the most dedicated I've met. Maryann Redford, Sangeeta Bhargava, Antonello Punturieri, Peyvand Ghofrani, and Karen Bienstock are marvels. I'm awed by your professionalism, your ability to ask hard questions, and your unfailing optimism that the work is making the world a better place.

Deep thanks to Janet Wittes for your generous forward, for your openness, and for embodying the claim that the best teachers are the most eager learners.

My colleagues and friends at Kent State University and NEOMED have been invaluable. Bioethicists Kimberly Garchar and Julie Aultman helped

clarify why this project matters. Philosophy Department colleagues Deborah C. Smith and Gina Zavota appreciated, and humored, enthusiasm for
an area of philosophy well outside their own. My chair, Michael Byron,
continues to support my work in whatever shape it takes. Good friends
across Kent State University—Susan Roxburgh, Tammy Clewell, and Mark
Bracher—always asked after my work and listened to countless monologues
about data safety monitoring. Your interest in my work has been unending.
Dear friends no longer at Kent State include Linda Williams, Wendy Shih,
Ronald Corthell, and Laura Bartolo. Tim Patrick assisted in compiling the
index; I am grateful for your hard work. I also thank Kent State University
for its continuing support of faculty research, including granting the Faculty Professional Improvement Leave that gave me time to work on this
project.

Friendship from Doris Kadish and Wendy Binder contributes to my flourishing in this life. Doris's mentorship has been invaluable; thank you for
reading and critiquing my work and for being the person I hope to be one
day. Wendy, my dearest friend of over forty years, I am stronger for your
strength.

MIT Press has been excellent. From day one, Phil Laughlin engaged this
project as if he knew it was valuable, unrelenting in the quest to bring it
to fruition. Haley Biermann is a boundless source of information. MIT's
editorial staff has been meticulous. Somewhere out there are a handful of
anonymous reviewers whose feedback made this book better. Thank you.

You cannot choose your family, but you can get damn lucky in having
the right one. Laurie is the best sister one could ever hope for—the greatest
ally, the strongest cheerleader, and as proud of me as I am of her. I'm grateful for the support of Todd, Starr, Michael, Susan, Shayna, Bruce, Karen,
Didi, and Sudeep. It is comforting to reflect on the fact that each of you
know how proud my parents would be of me. Having lost them both, your
support means all the more.

Finally, I am so grateful for my husband, Gene. His willingness to read
my writing, engage in discussions of data safety monitoring, and toler-
ate long stretches of my endless work can never be repaid. He is brilliant,
knowledgeable, and creative, and he is the best life partner I could have
ever imagined. I am staggered by my good fortune every day.

Introduction

Before anyone boards the plane, long before it taxis away from the gate, the preflight inspection begins. The instruments are checked, the flaps on the wings are tested, and the landing gear is assessed. The plane passes its inspection and is deemed worthy to transport its crew and passengers. But *once the plane takes flight*, that is when a circumstance might emerge that alters the flight plan or puts passengers in danger. Turbulence might require the Fasten Seatbelt sign to be turned on. A storm could necessitate a climb to bypass threatening weather. The runways at the destination airport may be obstructed, and the plane may have to circle until it is cleared to land. Even if the plane's preflight inspection determined it was in perfect condition before takeoff, without vigilance during the journey and without attending to the factors that may lead to a necessary course correction, the travelers could be in jeopardy.

The preboarding inspection is essential, of course, but a great deal of effort to avoid danger happens after the plane takes flight. *Only once a journey begins* do the greatest challenges emerge to keeping people safe.

* * *

In 2006, I was invited to serve on data safety monitoring boards (DSMBs) as a clinical ethicist and patient advocate for two projects sponsored by the National Institutes of Health (NIH). DSMBs are the committees that both recommend approval of clinical research before it commences and, more significantly, regularly meet to evaluate the data while the research is taking place, although not every trial that engages human participants is overseen by a DSMB. DSMBs are akin to the pilots, crew, and ground control who monitor the flight after it takes off, making sure that the journey is safe throughout. I would meet alongside handpicked experts every six months to pore over the data, ensuring that the studies remained on track and that the human participants were adequately protected. Serving on these two DSMBs opened doors to a decade-and-a-half engagement with data safety monitoring for the NIH, university-sponsored research, and private industry and collaboration with impressive scientists across the United States. DSMB work, coupled with engagement in reviewing grants and service on institutional review boards (IRBs), afforded me an extensive view of the regulatory landscape—from the inception of clinical research through its execution and completion. The experience of data safety monitoring has taught me a great deal, initiating a reevaluation of the role of ethicists in protecting human research participants.[1]

This book examines some of what I've learned about the DSMB dimension of research oversight and serves as a tool for potential DSMB members and others interested in bioethics in general. The lens through which I'm viewing DSMB work is primarily my participation in monitoring several NIH-sponsored trials. Each institute within the NIH has its own regulations detailing the operation and advisability of DSMB involvement. As such, the NIH trials used to illustrate ethical issues confronted by DSMBs aren't representative of every DSMB interaction—especially industry-sponsored trials. This book isn't meant to be an exhaustive assessment of DSMB issues. Given that there aren't other books that focus exclusively on a bioethics perspective on data safety monitoring, this volume is meant as the first in what I hope to be a larger conversation.[2] The small number of book-length discussions on DSMB work have focused on DSMB operational policy as well as statistical considerations. Rather than prioritizing operational policy or a statistical approach to DSMB deliberations, this volume examines the *bioethical* dimensions of DSMB work. Researchers whose work is scrutinized by DSMBs may learn what ethicists find important when monitoring trials. Those building their own safety monitoring processes from the ground up can learn from my experiences and anticipate the kind of concerns that ethicists raise. This book may be a tool to address an ongoing issue for DSMBs—"the underrepresentation of bioethicists"—by serving as a roadmap for bioethicists who need training in the monitoring arena (Department of Health and Human Services Office of Inspector General 2013, 12). As Eckstein, Rid, Kamuya, and Shah (2021, 2128) contend, "DSMBs lack substantive ethical guidance for the value judgments they are often required to make," which is why they call for "specific guidance on the ethical issues faced by DSMBs" (2129). For those who don't have data safety monitoring in their future, this book will nonetheless share insights about the ethical thinking that goes into monitoring clinical trials and the complex ethical deliberations that keep research participants safe.

Prior to DSMB work, I was an IRB aficionado, serving on three different IRBs and chairing two over the course of my career. IRBs are research ethics boards whose primary responsibility is to approve research on humans before studies begin. IRBs are akin to the ground crew, doing a final inspection before the plane is ready to take off and ensuring that everything is in place before the flight begins. Seeing firsthand the best IRBs could do and the ways in which they fell short, I was aware of the strengths and weaknesses of the IRB system. I've not abandoned IRBs—I still serve on one—or their importance. But my work on both IRBs and DSMBs has taught me that while each serve their purposes, a significant portion of the work protecting human subjects often falls to DSMBs. DSMBs oversee research projects as they unfold; they are the first to see the impact of the research investigation on human participants, and they are and entrusted with the welfare of those volunteers. Once the research journey begins, they are the ones who monitor the project and recommend a change of course if needed. However, even with all their importance, DSMBs are often comparatively unrecognized in the bioethics community. It is as if most of the attention and instruction went to the ground crew, and little attention went to the training of the flight crew.

Understanding what DSMBs do begins by examining the history of the more familiar system for the protection of human research participants: the IRB.[3] Chapter 1 begins by looking at the IRB system, how it evolved, and where it is today. IRB evaluation is primarily focused on research protocols before research begins, with only a precursory evaluation of projects while the research is in process. What is the evolution of ethical protections such that *historically a greater emphasis has been on the ethics of protocols even before they are initiated*? This history is examined so that the focus on review before a study begins can be best understood. The IRB system has undergone significant change in the last few years, owing to concerns that it was cumbersome and ineffective. Chapter 1 continues by reviewing discontents with the IRB system. A significant overhaul of the IRB system was finalized in June 2018 and went into effect in January 2019.[4] Some of the changes streamline the IRB process and allow IRBs to better focus their energies on human participant protections. But the IRB's primary focus, even in light of these new regulations, is on the ethical protections in place *before research even starts*. DSMBs, however, don't restrict their evaluation to trials only before they commence, but also while they are in process. DSMBs are chosen to ensure that clinical research is ethical both before the project starts and, importantly, *as the project continues*.

Chapter 1 proceeds with a discussion of the history of data monitoring as well as the policies that inform the mission and membership of DSMBs. The emergence of DSMBs is traced back to the Greenberg Report, commissioned by scientists not only to prevent the initiation of unethical research but also to ensure that ongoing research remained ethical. Unlike IRBs, there are no uniform policies that dictate the proceedings or processes of DSMBs—different organizations diverge on the specifics. Each NIH institute has its own policy on the composition and duties of DSMBs and when they are required. The Food and Drug Administration (FDA) has its own guidance document, "Guidance for Clinical Trial Sponsors: Establishment and Operation of Clinical Trial Data Monitoring Committees." For those interested in an international perspective, the World Health Organization has its "Operational Guidelines for the Establishment and Functioning of Data Safety Monitoring Boards." The latter two are merely "guidance" documents; not every committee adheres to these recommendations. To further complicate matters, monitoring committees are referred to using disparate terminology. The FDA's guidelines, the DAMOCLES study group, and the European Medicines Agency reference "DMCs," or data monitoring committees.[5] Some institutes located in the NIH reference "DSMCs," data safety monitoring committees. Elsewhere, the acronym "IDMC," for independent data monitoring committee, is used. Throughout this book, I'll be using the acronym "DSMB," except when directly engaging the policies that use other acronyms. While there are differences among the terms that reference these oversight committees, as well as their guiding documents, there are some commonalities all DSMBs share. The core missions and responsibilities of DSMBs are reviewed. Finally, to illustrate the importance of the work of DSMBs, chapter 1 concludes with an examination of a case in which a DSMB didn't succeed in protecting either participants or future patients. The Vioxx trials present an example of a failure of independence and transparency that resulted in the approval of a drug that had to be withdrawn from the market. This was a case in which autonomous and informed monitoring might have made a difference, thus demonstrating the value of what DSMBs add to research protections.

Chapters 2–5 in this volume examine unique challenges I encountered firsthand, each viewed through the lens of an NIH-sponsored clinical trial on whose DSMB I served. These clinical trials are invoked to illustrate some of the ethical dilemmas that emerge in DSMB work. These chapters include both an in-depth examination of some of the work that DSMBs do and real-world case studies of challenging aspects of safety monitoring. While the experiences and ethical challenges discussed do not exhaust the range of issues confronted by DSMBs, they are a starting point in understanding a DSMB's unique work.

Chapter 2 examines what an ethicist brings to the DSMB table, as illustrated by a trial in pulmonary medicine, the STRIVE-IPF trial. The STRIVE-IPF trial was a phase II study initiated to test a novel therapy for a fatal disease—acute exacerbations of idiopathic pulmonary fibrosis. In addition to clinical specialists and biostatisticians, some DSMBs include a bioethicist who specializes in clinical trials, although there is no consensus as to whether an ethicist is recommended on each DSMB. Ethicists are uniquely trained in the ethical foundations of human subject research and the policies that govern that research. The chapter begins by looking at the role of a DSMB ethicist as an expert in ethics policy. Ethicists may also be asked to serve as the voice of participants, as a participant or patient advocate. The scope and limits of this "patient advocate" role are examined in detail. In addition to being an expert in ethical policy, or a patient advocate, the ethicist also brings an outsider's perspective that can occasion scientific experts on the DSMB to look at data in new ways. This new way of looking at the data is the focus of the next section of chapter 2. The STRIVE-IPF trial was one such opportunity—a trial in which a "typical ethicist" question gave a DSMB biostatistician the opportunity to reconfigure the trial's data presentation for fellow members. This examination of the trial data reassured the DSMB that human participants were adequately protected and that the balance of potential benefits over potential risks continued to be positive. The ethicist at the DSMB table serves several roles, all of which contribute to the protection of human participants.

In some cases, DSMBs give their assessment of trials to sponsors before the trials start, considering if the potential benefits of the trial outweigh the

potential risks, as well as an assessment that the informed consent document and informed consent process convey the possible risks. Chapter 3
uses the cultivated autologous limbal epithelial cell (CALEC) study as a way
of understanding the challenges inherent in measuring these risks, as well
as the way informed consent evolves as risk profiles evolve. CALEC study
participants were enrolled after experiencing trauma to one of their eyes.
The participants then received a transplant of tissue from their healthy
eye to the damaged eye, called a CALEC transplant. The primary endpoint
of the study was to investigate if CALEC surgery was feasible. This transplant
could prove to be one of many steps, in the best-case scenario, to restoring at
least partial sight to each participant's damaged eye. The DSMB in the CALEC
study came to an important realization about the complexities of evaluating
possible risks and benefits in the CALEC trial, illustrating the intricate nature
of these assessments. The first section of chapter 3 examines the complexities of measuring risks in a study, as illustrated by the CALEC trial. Once the
DSMB was assured that the novel risks of CALEC were outweighed by the
potential benefits of the study, the next step was to ensure that the informed
consent document appropriately reflected those risks. The second section
discusses how to communicate those possible risks to participants.

However, the DSMB review of informed consent documents and processes may not be limited to review at the beginning of a study; the DSMB
needs to make sure that the informed consent is accurate, even as new
information becomes available over the course of a study (Friedman and
Schron 2008). The chapter's third section looks at the DSMB's role in recommending alterations of consent forms as studies progress. Since the DSMB
reviews new data as they emerge, the DSMB also has the responsibility to
recommend informing participants if new data may affect participants'
choices to remain in a study. Chapter 3 concludes with an illustration of
the complexities facing DSMBs as risk profiles change and what this means
for informed consent. The calculations made by the DSMB to recommend
changes to informed consent are intricate and do not always warrant an
automatic revision of informed consent.

Chapter 4 examines one of the most significant responsibilities DSMBs
are charged with: recommending to study sponsors that a clinical trial be
stopped (Friedman and Schron 2008). Clinical trials can be stopped for several reasons, such as the failure to recruit a sufficient number of research

participants, the discovery of new information that affects the continuation of the trial, or a reason to believe that some participants face significant risk or harm, or significant benefit, by virtue of being in the study. The decision to stop a trial early must be weighed against the competing forces that argue in favor of a study continuing: amassing enough data to convince the clinical community of the findings as well as the fact that if a study is stopped early, the contributions of participants may have been for naught. The DRCR Retina Network undertook two studies, referred to as Protocols AG and AH, to examine a novel way of closing a macular hole, a small hole in the retina that could compromise vision. Protocols AG and AH were stopped early because of a significant ethical concern: The monitoring committee believed that the studies fell out of equipoise. Equipoise, in ordinary language, can be understood as the notion that each participant is neither advantaged nor disadvantaged by virtue of the treatment to which they are randomly assigned in a study. But even this ordinary language notion is the subject of spirited debate among bioethicists. Chapter 4 begins with an examination of the concept of *equipoise*, analyzing competing claims as to what *equipoise* means. The second section of chapter 4 addresses how equipoise should be evaluated and the role of DSMBs in evaluating equipoise in clinical trials. Finally, the third section of chapter 4 revisits Protocols AG and AH, case studies in the application of equipoise to recommend closing a clinical trial. There isn't a consensus in the bioethics community about what *equipoise* means, or whether it matters. Chapter 4 explores this concept in depth to better illustrate what is at stake in DSMB deliberations.

Chapter 5 begins with a discussion of the SIGHT trial, a trial designed to examine three possible treatments for ophthalmologic complications of idiopathic intercranial hypertension. Idiopathic intercranial hypertension can result in progressive vision loss. This three-arm trial was ultimately stopped early because of a lack of enrolled participants. The difficulty in recruiting participants in this study was a multifaceted problem. The discussion in chapter 5 isn't meant to provide a definitive history as to why the SIGHT trial was unsuccessful—no member of the DSMB or the research team, or study participant, has all the answers. But from the perspective of *this member* of the DSMB, it was clear early on that recruitment of participants in this study would be a challenge. Many of the SIGHT participants experienced intersectional disadvantages in health care. Chapter 5 begins by looking at the barriers to recruiting diverse populations for research and the role of DSMBs in making recommendations to researchers and study sponsors regrading protecting populations who already experience structural disadvantages.

Once the COVID-19 pandemic began, it seemed as if *all research partici-pants became disadvantaged in some ways*, and *all research goals* became more difficult to accomplish. Natural disasters such as the pandemic, or political or armed conflicts, can disrupt research activities. The next section in chapter 5 examines some of the challenges that emerged during the pandemic and the ways in which DSMBs were forced to quickly pivot to preserve participant safety and allow the continuation of clinical research. Some of the points raised in chapters 3 and 4 about risk and equipoise are reexamined; COVID-19 changed possible risk profiles for research in unexpected ways, poten-ially raising questions of equipoise. The distinct topics of chapters 2–5—what an ethicist brings to the table, how to evaluate risks, the imperative to maintain equipoise, protecting vulnerable participants—blend together as coordinated concerns for the DSMB. The last section of chapter 5 presents practica recommendations for DSMB members so that they can help foster successful projects, even in the face of research challenges.

There is an additional point about the discussion of the trials in chapters 2–5: All DSMB deliberations are confidential. The summaries of the research protocols at the beginning of chapters 2–5 are taken from publicly available resources, such as the clinicaltrials.gov database, or from publications about trial outcomes. The discussion of the lessons and ethical insights drawn from experiences reviewing these trials is my own.[6]

The final chapter is the most theoretical. Chapter 6 argues for the bioethical foundation that informs the work of DSMBs: *Since the ethic that guides clinical research is a consequentialist ethic*, the ethical assessment of clinical research is best executed *throughout the duration of a research protocol*. Restricting the bulk of ethical assessments to the time prior to initiation of the research protocol—the primary work of IRBs, not DSMBs—results in an incomplete ethical analysis. This incomplete ethical analysis is akin to doing a rigorous inspection of the plane before it takes off, but not taking care to monitor the safety of the aircraft once in flight. Two arguments are put forward for placing the work of DSMBs, and their recommendations to sponsors as to how to best keep trial participants safe, at the center of research ethics.

The first argument proceeds from the fact that while most human subjects research is understood to be governed by a principlist bioethical approach—incorporating four prima facie principles of respect for autonomy, beneficence, nonmaleficence, and justice—there are nonetheless conspicuous examples of clinical research in which autonomy takes a back seat to concerns about possible risks and benefits. The autonomy of human research participants, as protected by informed consent, is often assumed to be foundational in research ethics, but when required in scientific trials, we allow compromises in autonomy for the sake of serving the greater good. That greater good can come in the form of the possibility of direct benefits to research participants, but most often comes in the form of the possibility of aspirational benefits—benefits to future patients and the promotion of generalizable knowledge. Several examples of clinical research are examined in which the autonomy protections of informed consent are waived to promote the production of benefits and the minimization of harm. These examples include some cases of research on persons unable to offer informed consent, some research on persons in the military, some research conducted during certain public health emergencies, or emergent circumstances. While rare each of these cases is an example of clinical research in which autonomy protections are outweighed by considerations of beneficence and nonmaleficence. However, there are no ethical trials in which participants autonomously consent, but which are nonetheless designed with the expectation that the trials will *not result in production of any direct or aspirational benefit, as well as minimization of harm.* Hence, there is a notable asymmetry: *Autonomy can be overridden* in some cases by an expectation of production of benefits and minimization of harm, but autonomy *never* overrides the expectation of a *failure* to produce any benefit and minimize of harm. This asymmetry calls into question the principlist approach to research ethics.

This negative argument—that research ethics is not a principlist one—is the first prong in the larger argument about the ethic that guides human research. The second prong is to argue positively that human research is an enterprise that *is* focused on the production of benefits and the minimization of harms. This positive argument examines the nature of clinical trials and their ultimate objectives. It is concluded that human subjects research is a consequentialist enterprise.

This is not to diminish the role of informed consent in participant protection. Autonomy protections afforded by informed consent are essential to overwhelming instances of clinical research. However, those autonomy-based concerns are secondary to the consequentialist considerations that

drive research. Human research may need informed consent, as a best practice both to protect autonomy and to maximize those consequences. However, there is no mistaking that minimizing potential risks and promoting
potential benefits are the primary ethical concerns in human research not
the protection of autonomy or justice. The ethical orientation of clinical
research is fundamentally consequentialist.

The disadvantage of consequentialism is that it doesn't give anyone
a rest. Consequentialism means always having to be vigilant, perpetu-
ally reassessing the decision to ask human participants to volunteer their
time and health and continuously ensuring that the potential benefits of
research outweigh possible harms. If we are to be true to this consequentialist ethic, then we must focus the ethical assessment of clinical research
not just before a research project commences, but throughout its duration.
Rather than front-loading ethical evaluation at the IRB level, we should
increase the ethical evaluation during the entirety of human subject participation. That is the role of DSMBs.

A second argument for the consequentialist ethic that drives clinical
research stems from one of the ethical imperatives that guides DSMBs:
maintaining equipoise. As seen in chapter 4, maintaining equipoise was the
ethical requirement that resulted in the monitoring committee recommending early closure of Protocols AG and AH. Interestingly, the view that maintaining equipoise is an ethical imperative is not held universally among
bioethicists. Some prominent bioethicists have taken an anti-equipoise
stance, arguing that the embrace of equipoise is based on either a mistaken
conception of research ethics or a therapeutic misconception about the
nature of research itself. These arguments are examined in detail. However,
I argue that while these arguments may persuasively call into question the
role of equipoise at the commencement of a trial, the arguments do not
apply when considering trials *as they progress*. The importance of equipoise
as trials progress yields two important conclusions. First, it underscores that
research ethics is in fact a consequentialist enterprise, focused on weighing
potential benefits against possible harms to achieve the best consequences.
Second, it means that the field of bioethics needs to retrain its focus beyond
evaluating a trial at its inception (the primary work of IRBs) and examine
more seriously the work done to monitor studies in progress (the work of
DSMBs). The DSMB is a committee of experts who oversee the progress
of a trial, alongside unblinded statisticians, the sponsor who pays for the

trial and may be responsible for site visits to ensure proper conduct of the study, steering committees that may have primary responsibility of both initial study design as well as writing primary manuscripts, and medical monitors who examine the possible harms that participants may experience. The DSMB's recommendations, in light of their scientific, statistical, and ethical analysis, can determine if a study is modified, suspended, or halted altogether.

According to Paul G. Wakim and Pamela A. Shaw, "The current literature on clinical trial monitoring and DSMBs is fairly extensive. Some books, guidance documents, journal articles, and videos focus on the logistical and regulatory side of safety and data monitoring; some focus on the statistical aspect of data monitoring; such as interim analysis; and some discuss both aspects" (Wakim and Shaw 2018, 138). Even within the extensive literature, the discussion of the *ethical aspects* of data safety monitoring is curiously limited. Christine Grady, in a discussion of the ethics of both IRBs and DSMBs, comments, "Although the amount of attention given to DSMBs has grown enormously in recent years, there is a need for continued investigation into the best methods of safety monitoring" (Grady 2019, 43) The role of the *bioethicist* on the DSMB, bringing their ethical expertise to the hands-on work of monitoring clinical trials, hasn't been adequately explored. This book shows how one bioethicist's expertise on DSMBs was marshaled to protect human research participants in several NIH-sponsored trials, serving as a guide both to bioethicists and to those who will be working with bioethicists in the future. Those who are serving on DSMBs, who are reporting their data to DSMBs, or who are in the nascent stages of creating their own data monitoring framework will profit from an examination of the ethical considerations that guide DSMBs. My hope in sharing my experiences, and the ethical framework that guided my own deliberations, is that these lessons will be of value to those studying bioethics, to future DSMB members of all backgrounds, to the researchers who rely on DSMBs to help them conduct ethical studies, and to the human participants whose safety has been entrusted to us.

1 What Are Data Safety Monitoring Boards, and What Is Their Role?

There are two oversight committees charged to evaluate the ethical use of human participants. The first are institutional review boards, or IRBs. The second are data safety monitoring boards, alternately data and safety monitoring boards (DSMBs), also referred to as data monitoring committees (DMCs) or data safety monitoring committees (DSMCs). While both IRBs and DSMBs are designed to protect the interests of human research subjects, each has a distinct history, membership, and mission. It is instructive to first examine what may be the more familiar means of protecting human research participants, the IRB, to understand the role of DSMBs. After examining the history of the IRB, its charge, and some challenges facing the IRB system, the distinct role of the DSMB will become clear. While IRBs and DSMBs share some common tasks, DSMBs are distinct from IRBs in their history, in their membership, in being project- or discipline-specific, and in their deep engagement with clinical trials and comparative trial data as studies progress.

The Historical Evolution of IRBs: One Means to Protect Human Research Participants

A good portion of bioethicists' work on research ethics concerns the work of IRBs.[1] Every institution that receives federal money for their principal investigators' research is required to have an IRB, and private industry studies that are conducted independently of federal support routinely have their work evaluated by an IRB. For multisite clinical trials, the IRB that oversees research is the IRB with which the project principal investigator (PI) is affiliated. Each institution that recruits participants does not need protocols to be vetted by their own IRB, although for years, local IRB oversight was required of any project that recruited research participants from a given institution.

The policies governing the IRB system have their origins in the 1974 National Research Act (Porter and Koski 2008). Amy Davis and Elisa Hurley observe the Act was passed "in response to a series of well-publicized and egregious research abuses during the first two-thirds of the twentieth century" (Davis and Hurley 2014, 10). A similar impetus was the basis for the establishment of Congress's National Commission for the Protection of Human Subjects of Biomedical and Behavioral Research. The National Commission was created after news of the Tuskegee Syphilis Study broke in the popular press (Emanuel and Menikoff 2011). The National Commission's recommendations became the basis of the Common Rule (45CFR46) in 1981; these rules were extended to fourteen federal departments in 1991. At present, twenty different agencies follow the Common Rule guidance.[2] Hence, the name "Common Rule"—these are the *rules* governing the use of human participants that are *common* across multiple agencies. The Common Rule details IRB functions, operations, and review activities, including copious directives about who should serve on IRBs, informed consent documents, and the nature of the materials reviewed by IRBs before a study can be approved. Only once a study receives IRB approval may researchers interact with human participants.

Carol Levine observed that our system of human participant protection was "born in scandal and reared in protectionism" (Levine 1988, 167). Greg Koski quotes Levine and further elaborates on her claims. Koski recounts a litany of unethical research in the United States that is familiar to those schooled in the history of human research protections (Koski 2014, 342–343): Tuskegee, Willowbrook, the Jewish Chronic Disease Hospital, the human radiation studies—the research abuses cited above by Davis and Hurley in the first two-thirds of the twentieth century. Unfortunately, the research abuses did not end there. Additional scandals include the tragic fate of Jessie Gelsinger, a healthy voluntary research participant in a trial to test the mechanism for delivering a novel gene therapy. The mechanism was a virus that was supposed to carry and distribute the altered genes throughout the body. "The researcher, a leading figure in the new, much-hyped field of gene therapy, had suspected problems with the laboratory-altered virus, but continued to inject it into subjects anyway, including Jesse" (Klitzman 2015, 192). The fact that the PI stood to gain financially from the success of the trial was not disclosed on the informed consent document. Another example of misguided research is the tragic fate of Ellen Roche, a healthy voluntary research participant who became significantly ill within twenty-four hours of taking the drug hexamethonium in a 2001 trial, only to pass away a month later. The PI on the study was later found to have not reported that the first participant had developed adverse events (AEs) as a result of taking the drug. The PI had not sufficiently researched hexamethonium, including the fact that the Food and Drug Administration (FDA) had withdrawn the drug from the market. The fact that the drug was both experimental and that it had previously been withdrawn was not on the informed consent document (Klitzman 2015, 117–118). It is little wonder, given these cases of research misconduct, that "historically the promulgation of rules governing the conduct of human subjects research has been not evidence driven but scandal driven" (Sachs 2010, 13). Unsurprisingly, "the history of research ethics is frequently described as 'reactive'" (Wenner 2018, 25).

Koski cautions that invoking these cases may result in mistakenly predicating the protection of human participants on a belief that researchers are inherently unethical, with the guiding hypothesis being that the only thing standing between researchers and the wholesale abuse of human participants are IRBs and similar regulatory bodies. This uncharitable assumption is likely unwarranted. Alternative explanations exist beyond impugning the intention of researchers. Even without assuming the *researchers* are unethical, the history of research oversight is that regulations need to be in place because *unethical studies* were *unethical from the beginning*. As Henry Beecher states, "An experiment is ethical or not at its inception; it does not become ethical post hoc" (Beecher 1966, 372). The horror of the Tuskegee Syphilis Study isn't that the study became unethical during its course.[3] Given the lack of truly informed consent, the coercive nature of participation, the exploitive nature of participant recruitment, and the fact that the study yielded no new data that wasn't previously known about the progress of a terminal and contagious disease, the study was unethical from the start. The same can be said of Willowbrook, the Jewish Chronic Disease Hospital, the human radiation experiments, and the research that led to the senseless deaths of Jesse Gelsinger and Ellen Roche. Irrespective of the intentions of the researchers, all are examples of research that should not have been performed in the first place.

After the Common Rule was initially codified in 1981, it was revised, most recently in 2018. The 2018 revisions were enacted in part owing to studies that demonstrated IRBs weren't doing their job as well as they should. As stated by Davis and Hurley (2014, 11), "The IRB system has been described as inefficient, over-burdened, lacking expertise, obstructionist to research, and underfunded." One comprehensive analysis of the problems with the IRB system prior to the 2018 revisions was Lura Abbott and Christine Grady's 2011 review of forty-three articles that reported empirical data on IRB functioning in the United States. Their findings chronicle myriad discontents with the IRB system: extensive and inconsistent times to approval, variations in assessment of risk, idiosyncratic requests for changes to consent forms that do not further participant protections, and inconsistent application of the federal regulations. Some of these findings (Shah, et al. 2004; Silverman, Hull, and Sugarman 2001; Stair et al. 2001; Mansbach et al. 2007) were the impetus for disbanding the system of local control and consolidating IRB review to a single IRB.

Laura Stark's ethnographic research on IRBs lead her to claim that IRBs often drew inconsistent conclusions about multisite studies not based on inadequate Common Rule guidance, but instead "because IRB members develop site-specific 'local precedents' to work more quickly and to make consistent decisions over time" (Stark 2014, 184). Localizing the oversight of human research protections was not merely a way of "passing the buck," deferring responsibility for oversight from the federal government to multiple IRBs: "For the community representatives and the researchers supporting them, local control is a reasonable response to prior injustices and to an unfair convention giving researchers near absolute control over data and results" (Dresser 2008, 234). At the same time, local control contributed to more paperwork, longer review times, and idiosyncratic responses from IRBs. It is little wonder that multisite reviews yielded multisite conclusions. As Angus, Gordon, and Bauchner (2021) observe, "The structure of the US clinical research enterprise is vast and has never functioned as a single national coordinated system." Centralizing IRB review presumably would diminish the vastness and the bureaucracy that accompanies it. Further, "it has been argued that for the great majority of multisite studies, critical IRB functions, including those ensuring that risks are minimized and balanced by benefits and that research is scientifically valid, are not dependent on local factors that only a local IRB can assess" (Emanuel and Menikoff 2011,

1147). The 2018 move to centralized IRB reviews for multisite research projects has been a positive development.

Additional changes in the 2018 revisions to the Common Rule included an attempt to streamline informed consent documents, to include additional protections for data held in genetic repositories, and the refining of "exempt" research categories—research that is exempt from a review by the entire IRB. These internal changes haven't entirely addressed all the issues surrounding IRB effectiveness. A Government Accountability Office (GAO) report released in February 2023 found that reviews of IRBs have not been comprehensive, and processes for assessing IRB effectiveness have not been codified, despite repeated calls for action. While some organizations such as the Consortium to Advance Effective Research Ethics Oversight (AEREO) are available to take up these challenges, the IRB system remains open to concern (Fernandez Lynch, Hurley, and Taylor 2023).

The most recent revisions to the IRB system do not mark a departure from the assumption that the basic structure of research protections executed by IRBs—employing heavy scrutiny of research protocols before they are initiated—is the best ethical safeguard. Koski holds that it is time for a serious rethink of the current regulatory system: "Perhaps we can come to a realization that we have bred a new generation of investigators, better trained, more responsible, more willing to do the right thing not because they are required to do so by regulations but because it is the right thing to do" (Koski 2014, 345). The background assumption that researchers are ethically responsible—that they do not willfully plan unethical research, but occasionally benefit from an IRB's wisdom in modifying consent forms, recruitment strategies, and the like—is an idea whose time has come.

The IRB model assumed that the best way to keep human participants safe is by first engaging in the appropriate ethical oversight, after which research can commence. Is it correct that the best ethical protection for human research is scrutiny prior to the research taking place?

What IRBs Are Not Charged to Do

IRB review overwhelmingly concerns approval *prior to the commencement of a research study*. IRB scrutiny is focused primarily on informed consent documents, the informed consent process, recruitment of human participants, and the presumptive benefits and harms of the research project. The

working assumptions given this front-loaded scrutiny are 1) research studies require initial vetting by an IRB to determine that they are ethical, 2)
research studies that are initially vetted by the IRB as ethical will remain so,
unless 3) deviations from the IRB-approved protocol render the research no
longer ethical. Once a research study has been approved by the IRB, as long
as everything goes as planned, little has to be done to ensure the research
is ethical. This is a somewhat deontological perspective on ethical human
trials: If the rules or principles that are in place are adequately followed,
then the research is ethical. Deviate from the rules, and there may be a
problem. Stick to the script, and the research is ethical.

Stark, in her history and ethnography of IRBs (Stark 2012), holds a somewhat modified view: Stark argues that IRBs are governed primarily by *people*,
not by *policy*. According to Stark, it is the individuals on the IRB, and their
interpretation of policy, that guide the ethical use of human research participants. While this appears to be a more subjectivist account than most
ethicists would prefer, there is also a decidedly deontological slant to this
approach. Even if individual IRB members are the ones whose *interpretations of policies* ultimately determine the appropriate scope of human subject protections at a given institution, researchers must nonetheless follow
those policies as interpreted by IRB members. IRBs provide a checklist—one
that may be crafted with some local interpretation—that must be followed
for the research to be ethical. If all goes well, and the checklist is followed,
then the research is presumed ethical.

Given the observation that IRBs were crafted by history and policy to
scrutinize research primarily before it takes place, it is unsurprising that
there are few references in the Common Rule concerning review of research
after the research has begun. Per the Common Rule, "An IRB shall conduct
continuing review of research covered by this policy at intervals appropriate to the degree of risk, but not less than once per year" (§46.109e) The
IRB is charged with making sure that the research plan includes appropriate
data monitoring (§46.111(6)), although the IRB itself is not charged with
monitoring the data. The Common Rule does not detail how the data are
monitored, by whom, or what this monitoring entails. There is little guidance about how research projects maintain a positive balance of potential
benefits over risks once they are in progress: "As a consequence, there is a
great degree of variability in the manner in which IRBs carry out this important function" (Gordon, Sugarman, and Kass 1998, 4). IRBs have the power

to suspend or terminate a research protocol in which the researchers did not follow the IRB's recommendations, or which "has been associated with unexpected serious harm to subjects" (§46.113). The IRB is not charged with gathering the data regarding unexpected serious harm, only with acting in response to those data. Reportable protocol deviations and AE data are to be communicated to the IRB, but the systematic collection of efficacy or benefit data is not required. These brief mentions of monitoring once a project has commenced can be contrasted, for example, with the dozens of paragraphs that describe the requirements and documentation of informed consent (§46.116 and §46.117), or even the five paragraphs that detail IRB membership (§46.107).

The Common Rule's relative depreciation of continuing review, data monitoring, and attention to the ongoing assessment of potential risks and benefits of clinical research should not be viewed as an objection to the Common Rule's directives. The Common Rule and IRBs are *doing exactly what they have been charged to do*. Given the history in which IRBs emerged—a history of scandals in which the greatest violation was that *unethical research commenced at all*—it is no surprise that IRB purview is almost exclusively focused on research protocols before they start.

Data Safety Monitoring Boards: A Distinct History, a Distinct Mission

DSMBs have a different origin story from IRBs: less well-established structures and a different focus in their shared effort to protect human research participants.

Several commenters trace the history of DSMBs to the Greenberg Report, written in 1967, commissioned by the National Heart Institute (NHI) (Gordon, Sugarman, and Kass 1998; DeMets, Furberg, and Friedman 2006). The NHI, later named the NHLI (National Heart Lung Institute) and most recently the NHLBI (National Heart Lung and Blood Institute), initiated a trial in 1965 referred to as the Coronary Drug Project (CDP), comparing five drugs and a placebo in 8,341 participants across fifty-three sites. Given the complexity of the large multisite CDP, the NHI recognized the necessity of organizing a policy board that would provide oversight of some aspects of the study. The Greenberg Report, named after its chairperson, Bernard Greenberg, presented a set of recommendations for what were referred to as "cooperative studies"—studies in which researchers from multiple institutions worked using a single protocol to collaboratively answer research questions. Among the recommendations for a "separately funded" committee that could maintain independence when evaluating the project were as follows:

> A Policy Board or Advisory Committee of senior scientists, experts in the field of the study but not data-contributing participants in it, is almost essential for a large complex cooperative project. Such a group can review the overall plan, make recommendations on any possible changes (including changes in protocol and operating procedures), adjudicate controversies that may develop, and advise the National Heart Institute on such matters as the addition of new participants or the dropping of nonproductive units. (Heart Special Project Committee 1988, 142–143)
>
> It is natural that the members of the review committee, being experts in many disciplines, should call upon their own experience and think of various ways in which the study might be modified and perhaps improved. (Heart Special Project Committee 1988, 144)
>
> Regular annual reports to both the review group and the National Heart Council would also serve to keep members up to date in regard to progress. They should be prepared by the Chairman of the study in cooperation with the Director of the Coordinating Center and the Executive Committee, and should be comprehensive delineations of the current status of the project. Such reports serve another purpose well, in that they can permit early detection of unforeseen weaknesses or problems in the study. It might then be possible to institute remedial measures before major difficulties develop. (Heart Special Project Committee 1988, 145)
>
> A mechanism must be developed for early termination if unusual circumstances dictate that a cooperative study should not be continued. Such action might be contemplated if the accumulated data answer the original question sooner than anticipated, if it is apparent that the study will not or cannot achieve its stated aims, or if scientific advances since initiation render continuation superfluous. This is obviously a difficult decision that must be based on careful analysis of past progress and future expectation. (Heart Special Project Committee 1988, 146)

The advice offered in the Greenberg Report was taken up in 1968, when the CDP Policy Board recommended that a safety monitoring committee be formed to review CDP data (DeMets, Furberg, and Friedman 2006). The NHI model was ultimately adopted for all NHI studies. Subsequently, the Office for Extramural Research established a committee on clinical trial monitoring, which affirmed that "all trials, even those that pose little likelihood of harm, should consider an external monitoring body" (National Institutes of Health 1998). Another landmark set of recommendations are those put forward by the DAMOCLES (Data Monitoring Committees: Lessons, Ethics,

Statistics) Study Group, commissioned by the UK's National Health Service to "investigate the processes of monitoring accumulating trial data and to identify ways of increasing the likelihood that DMCs make good decisions" (DAMOCLES 2005, 711). Per the National Institutes of Health's (NIH) 1998 guidelines, the level of monitoring should be commensurate with the perceived degree of risk. Some projects may require merely ongoing monitoring by the PI, an informal body, or a steering committee. Others will demand an independent DSMB.

Unlike IRBs, which were born from research scandals surrounding projects that should never have been initiated, DSMBs have their origins in less trying circumstances. For one, *the NHI itself* commissioned the Greenberg Report, anticipating that there may be problems in running a large multisite trial. DSMBs were created in collaboration with researchers, not imposed from outside to police researchers. If anything, the Greenberg model may be criticized from a contemporary perspective for too close a collaboration with the researchers. The policy board was conceived in the Greenberg Report as working with the trial's steering committee. Per the above, reports were to be "prepared by the Chairman of the study in cooperation with the Director of the Coordinating Center and the Executive Committee," a collaboration that today would be viewed as a conflict of interest, potentially compromising the objectivity of DSMB assessments. While DSMB work has evolved from the Greenberg model, the fact that the NHI itself initiated a monitoring process is significant. Unlike IRBs, whose mandate was imposed from outside, the NHI recognized the value of continuing oversight, owing to the complexity of the CDP. IRBs were formed to create rules that might prevent unethical research from starting—hence Koski's observations that much of research oversight emerged from a fraught history. DSMBs, however, were formed to create surveillance for studies that were ethical when they commenced but *required oversight as they continued* to ensure they remained ethical.

The proactive response of the NHI can be contrasted with the reactive response that created IRBs. IRBs emerged because researchers made mistakes; DSMBs emerged because researchers wanted to ensure that they *didn't* make mistakes. The upside of this distinct history is that in many cases, DSMBs have a less adversarial relationship with researchers. DSMBs comprise experts in the field in which the research takes place, but who don't have conflicts of interest such as engagement with the research they are monitoring or a vested interest in the outcome of the trial (Department of Health and Human Services, Office of Inspector General 2013). "A DSMB plays a unique role in a clinical trial, for by design its members have no reason, financial or intellectual, to prefer one result over another" (Wittes et al. 2007, 229). DSMB members can been seen as well-informed, objective experts.

As Stark observes, IRBs were initially "place based"—each institution had its own IRB, taking into account local precedent in forming conclusions about ethical research, with the IRB reviewing any and all research that happened to be taking place at that institution. For this reason, members of a given IRB would unlikely be potential collaborators on the research projects they evaluate. DSMBs are "protocol based," mustering the expertise of individuals who could just as well be doing the research they happen to be monitoring. While this means that DSMB membership needs to be carefully crafted, so as to avoid conflicts of interest, it also means each DSMB member comes to the table with unique expertise in the projects they monitor. Wittes et al. (2007), for example, in discussing the experience of the DSMB for the Women's Health Initiative Clinical Trials, recount that during the trial, emerging data indicated that knowledge in the area of dementia was warranted. As a result, several years into the trials, the sponsor added two DSMB members with expertise in dementia. The DSMB initially didn't include members with this background, but it became clear that monitoring the safety of participants required additional know-how.

There is no single policy that informs DSMB composition or activities across the NIH, FDA, or industry. Even the question regarding when a DSMB is required to monitor a study is a subject about which there is no universal agreement. The FDA's nonbinding recommendations for DMCs are codified in their "Guidance for Clinical Trial Sponsors: Establishment and Operation of Clinical Trial Data Monitoring Committees" (2006). The FDA's recommendations note that increased collaboration among government agencies and private sponsors has resulted in an increased use of data monitoring committees than in the past, although the *legal requirement* for monitoring of FDA-sponsored trials is currently limited only to emergent research studies that include a waiver of informed consent, per 21 CFR 50.24(a)(7)(iv); these studies are discussed in greater detail in chapter 6. The FDA's recommendations note that "all clinical trials require safety monitoring, but not all trials require monitoring by a formal committee that may be external to the trial organizers, sponsors, and investigators" (U.S. Department of Health and Human Services 2006, 3). The FDA notes that DMCs are typically indicated for "large, multisite studies that evaluate treatments intended to prolong life or reduce risk of a major adverse health outcome," but not all clinical research requires a DMC (U.S. Department of Health and Human Services 2006, 3). The FDA also claims that DMCs "are not usually warranted in early studies such as Phase 1 or early Phase 2 studies," although even then there are possible exceptions based on expectations of safety and degree of risk (U.S. Department of Health and Human Services 2006, 23). The NIH requires all phase III multisite trials it sponsors that may pose risk to participants be monitored by a DSMB (Department of Health and Human Services, Office of Inspector General 2013). Cairns, Hallstrom, and Held (2001, 156) state, "A DSMC seems essential when a trial has the power to detect statistically significant differences in tangible human outcomes," when risks are unpredictable, or when the therapy under study is known to have severe risks. The European Medicines Agency (EMA) (2005, 4) advises, "When it comes to the decision whether a DMC should be set up or not aspects such as indication, study endpoint(s), study duration as well as study population should be taken into consideration. Also, the available knowledge about a drug might trigger the need for a DMC." The EMA goes on to recommend the use of a DMC in most trials for life-threatening conditions, for pediatric populations, when participants are at risk of harm, or when interim analyses are expected to yield possible modifications in study design. However, they also caution that in some cases, establishing a DMC could slow down a study and may be contraindicated. Grady's summary of the first edition of Ellenberg, Fleming, and DeMets (first edition 2002, second edition 2019) is that "DSMBs are usually required for late phase clinical trials, randomized controlled trials testing drugs, biologics, devices or surgical procedures, complex and/or multicenter trials, or studies involving an intervention with anticipated concern about safety or risk or study participants who might need additional protection" (Grady 2019, 40).

The DAMOCLES study group noted that with the exception of the 2002 edition of Ellenberg, Fleming, and DeMets, "little explicit guidance has been published" on standard operating procedures or charters for data monitoring committees (DAMOCLES 2005, 711). Lisa Eckstein concurs, observing "a paucity of legal or ethical frameworks governing these Boards' composition or operation, or their relationship with other actors with monitoring responsibility" (Eckstein 2015, 81). Hence, DAMOCLES issued their own recommendations in an attempt to close this gap. Some of the institutes within the NIH have their own policies regarding DSMBs, and some regulations are institute-wide. One drawback that emerges from the origin of DSMBs is that "there are no broadly accepted guidelines or regulations that govern [DSMB's] structure or operation" (Gordon, Sugarman, and Kass 1998, 1). There was no hearing convened in the wake of a scandal that precipitated DSMB oversight, no National Commission, and no "Common Rule" that guides DSMB membership or responsibilities. Some have claimed that the lack of uniformity is a strength and not a weakness, as it avoids classifying clinical trials, for example, "generically into those that do and those that do not need a DSMB, without knowing the details of each trial" (Wakim and Shaw 2018, 129). Here, the contrast with IRBs is stark. The Common Rule presents detailed discussion of eight categories of research that are exempt from IRB oversight (45 CFR §46.104), whereas there is no uniform policy as to when a DSMB is required.

There is agreement that "the main function of the DSMB is to provide continuous evaluation of the accumulating trial data that researchers, usually blinded to emerging trial data, cannot undertake. These interim analyses examine both efficacy and safety" (Gordon, Sugarman, and Kass 1998, 2). DSMBs have responsibility to "ensure [a clinical trial] does not compromise the safety of its participants" and to "ensure data integrity" (Wakim and Shaw 2018, 127). Among the activities DSMBs may perform toward these ends are recommending approval of projects before they are initiated, including reviewing balance of possible risks over possible benefits, the study methodology, and the statistical analysis plan including the "data shells" that reflect the categories of data and how they will be reported to the DSMB; reviewing the informed consent process and documents; holding regular meetings while the study is in progress to review newly published information that may affect the study, monitoring of recruitment, retention, and dropouts of participants, adherence of different sites to the protocol and protocol deviations, interim data, AEs, and serious adverse events (SAEs), including possible formal interim analyses for efficacy or futility; recommending or approving modifications of study methodology, the statistical analysis plan, or informed consent; and making formal recommendations to approve continuation, modification, temporarily halting, or terminating the trial. Jay Herson observes that committees in "NIH-sponsored trials are usually involved in trial design, sample size requirements, data analysis methods, data quality, publications policy, investigator evaluation, and so on, in addition to efficacy and safety review" (Herson 2017, 4), which in some cases is a more extensive role for monitors than in trials with other sponsorships. Calis et al. reported that a representative group of data monitoring committee members thought that committees should have a limited role in designing trials, as such involvement could contribute to bias in the studies. At the same time, committee members were in favor of "hav(ing) the opportunity to review the study protocol and offer suggestions before the study is launched" (2017, 61–62). DeMets and Friedman argue that one of the advantages in having a DSMB in place before a study commences is that "the DSMB may have some constructive suggestions regarding the design which are difficult to incorporate once the trial is underway" (2006, 206).

DSMBs meet both in open sessions with the researchers and sponsors of the trial to discuss trial progress and in closed sessions that exclude researchers so that the DSMB can examine data to which the researchers do not yet have access. Some DSMBs have closed executive sessions, which exclude researchers as well as any representative from the sponsor, with no one present other than the DSMB members (Wittes et al. 2007). These closed sessions afford the DSMB the opportunity to discuss the quality of the reports compiled by an independent statistical reporting group so that the DSMB can be assured it has quality data, allowing it to perform its function well. Both open and closed session data are compiled by study statisticians. Closed session meetings may include statisticians who are unblinded to the data. After each DSMB meeting, both open session and closed session reports are issued, including the minutes of the meeting. The open session report should not include any information that reveals comparative results. The investigators and sponsors have access to the open session report only, as the closed session report may contain findings that would bias the researchers or sponsors. The open session report may recommend continuing the study as is, changing the study or the consent procedures, temporarily halting the study pending further information, or stopping a study altogether. In many cases, the study sponsor is responsible for conveying those minutes to the IRB overseeing the study, letting the IRB know of the DSMB's recommendations to continue a study, to modify a study, or to terminate a study. In addition to regularly scheduled meetings,

DSMB meetings can be convened on an emergency, as-needed basis. For example, if evidence of a significant disruption in balance of risks over benefits emerges, or major protocol deviations signal that participants may be at greater risk than was formerly known, then a previously unscheduled meeting may be in order. While many of these procedures are laid out in the guidance documents from the NIH, the FDA, DAMOCLES, and other sources, it should be stressed that those are mere *guidance* documents; there is no legal requirement that monitoring committees adhere to the above strictures.

One way in which IRBs and DSMBs may be similar is that both exert some level of control over research studies—shaping the processes of the study, the interaction with participants, and the analyses. Beyond the concerns cited above about the idiosyncratic evaluations of IRBs, there are also concerns that IRBs have too much power—power to recommend changes not only to the consent process and forms but also to research methodologies, in the name of protecting human research participants. Might the same objection be made about DSMBs, that they wield too much power when they recommend changes to a clinical trial's design, statistical analysis, consent process and forms? DSMBs have even more power than that, insofar as they can communicate directly with a study's sponsor or steering committee to recommend halting a study in progress if the study demonstrates efficacy, futility, or other types of failures (such as a failure to recruit participants). Eckstein's recommendations for greater integration between IRB and DSMB oversight of trials emerges from her concerns about "DSMB's sweeping discretion in deciding whether and when to recommend that a trial should be terminated or amended," given "DSMB's monopoly over emerging trial data" (Eckstein 2015, 81). This concern about the power of DSMBs is tempered slightly by the fact that the DSMB's power is merely recommendatory. Per the DAMOCLES study group, it is important that data monitoring committees serve in this type of "advisory rather than executive function"—*recommending rather than mandating* a particular course of action to the sponsor or steering committee, so that it is clear that the sponsor, not the data monitors, have ultimate responsibility over the trial (DAMOCLES 2005, 713). Recommendations have been made to include indemnification language in DSMB charters to ensure that this recommendatory responsibility does not expose DSMB members to legal liability (DeMets et al. 2004). However, even in this advisory role, DSMBs have the power to shape the course of trials. The bioethics literature is rife with complaints that IRBs have too much power (Stark 2012; Briggs 2022). Why aren't there similar concerns about DSMBs?

One possible answer is that, per the above discussion, DSMBs have merely *recommendatory* power, whereas IRBs wield *regulatory* power. However, while this might appear to be the easy answer, my inclination is that this distinction is insufficient to explain disparate views of DSMBs and IRBs by researchers. Regulatory power alone doesn't always yield respect. If it did, then children would respect the police more than their peers, and citizens would respect the IRS more than community bankers. While the more powerful entities may engender fear, and thus complaints, they don't necessarily command respect. However, these analogies prove illuminating, as peers and community bankers have two properties that promote respect. First, they are well known and familiar. Second, by virtue of the fact that they don't wield the might of the police or the IRS, it falls to them to be persuasive via familiarity or argument, not force.

Rather than attribute the greater number of complaints about IRBs, contra DSMBs, to the greater regulatory power wielded by IRBs, two additional possibilities emerge. The first is that IRBs have simply received far more attention from bioethicists than DSMBs. There are more books, articles, conferences, professional organizations, and the like devoted to IRBs. IRBs are an easier target because everyone knows where to look for them. This may be a dissatisfying answer, in that it only occasions the next question: *Why are* IRBs more prominent in the bioethics literature than DSMBs? Here I can only speculate. One possible reason is that there are simply more IRBs than DSMBs. Nearly every hospital and university—certainly those that are doing their own research—have their own IRB. A 2023 GAO report found the Department of Health and Human Services oversees approximately 2,300 IRBs in the United States (GAO, 2023). Unlike IRBs, DSMBs are typically only used in a subset randomized clinical trials, and even then, as stated above, there are no uniform requirements for DSMB oversight across NIH, FDA, and industry. There are simply *fewer* DSMBs than IRBs. With less exposure comes less scrutiny. Academics studying the ethics of human research have less exposure to the inner workings of DSMBs than IRBs.

A second theory addressing why DSMBs have received less pushback than IRBs is more nuanced and goes back to both the individuals who compose the respective committees and their respective histories. Since IRBs are site specific, they comprise individuals who are affiliated with a particular institution. Prior to the 2018 revision of the Common Rule, all multisite projects had to be reviewed by the IRB from each institution that recruited participants. FDA regulations state that all "clinical investigations that are intended to support applications for research or marketing permits for FDA-regulated products" need to be reviewed by a registered IRB (21 CFR §56.106); industry seeking FDA approval for drugs or medical devices must obtain IRB approval. Since the 2018 Common Rule revision, each multisite project needs to be reviewed by only a single IRB, where the IRB is a standing committee that reviews all research that originates at that institution. The FDA offered its own guidance on centralized IRB review in 2006.[4] IRBs are not convened as experts in a particular area. Additionally, owing to the history that created the IRB system—a history of project research that should never have been started—IRBs carry the stigma of "policing" research. This history creates the impression that IRBs are a pool of individuals *who aren't necessarily well-acquainted with the nuances of each protocol* but are there primarily to prevent researchers from making ethical mistakes.

Each DSMB, however, has a membership chosen for specific projects or specific research groups. For this reason, DSMBs comprise specialists in the area of research they oversee. Researchers may perceive members of the DSMB as their peers. Open sessions of DSMB meetings, with open session minutes shared with the sponsors who subsequently share with researchers, mean that researchers know the members of the DSMB, and vice versa. The result may be that DSMBs have, or are at least perceived to have, greater expertise in the trials they monitor than IRB members. Second, in light of the history of DSMBs, they emerged less as *police* and more as *partners* in the research enterprise. DSMBs thus have more in common with peer groups, or community bankers—equals in expertise, making recommendations based on insights about a trial's data and informed argument. DSMBs may wield comparable power as IRBs, but that power may be viewed as more legitimate.

A Case Study on the Importance of DSMBs: Lessons from the Vioxx Trials

One way to demonstrate the importance of DSMB work is to examine a case that sheds light on the centrality of the DSMB's role in protecting research participants as well as future cohorts of patients. A prominent example is the case of rofecoxib, known by its brand name Vioxx, developed by Merck to treat rheumatoid arthritis. Vioxx was approved by the FDA in 1998 on the basis of nine studies; however, those "nine studies were generally small, had short treatment periods, enrolled patients at low risk of cardiovascular disease, and did not have a standardised procedure to collect and adjudicate cardiovascular outcomes" (Krumholz, Ross, Presler, and Egilman 2007, 120). In other words, in lieu of procedures to collect and adjudicate cardiovascular outcomes, the risks to participants may not have been adequately monitored.

After approval, Merck commenced a larger study of Vioxx, the Vioxx Gastrointestinal Outcomes Research (VIGOR) study. Even though Vioxx had FDA approval, the goal of the VIGOR study was to establish a safety profile that might allow Vioxx to be prescribed for a larger number of indications. A great deal of money was at stake in making Vioxx available to a larger patient population. "The study of over 8000 patients was initiated without a standard operating procedure for collecting information on cardiovascular events and without a cardiologist on the data safety monitoring board" (Krumholz et al. 2007, 120). The chair of the VIGOR DSMB was arguably in a conflict of interest after having received a $70,000 consulting contract from Merck. The DSMB, in two separate interim analysis meetings, saw evidence in one treatment group of a higher risk of death or serious cardiovascular events. Rather than recommending halting the study temporarily or indefinitely, the DSMB recommended an additional analysis plan to follow those cardiac AEs.

Once the final results of the study were in, it was indisputable that Vioxx caused elevated cardiac AEs, although participants in the Vioxx arm experienced fewer gastrointestinal bleeds, and the deaths across both arms appeared comparable. The DSMB might have at this point recommended that the publications of the VIGOR results truthfully communicate the risk/benefit profile of Vioxx. While DSMBs don't have an active role in writing publications after a study, they may be charged with review of final manuscripts, especially primary manuscripts, to ensure the data and conclusions are accurately represented (DeMets and Ellenberg, 2016). The publication of the VIGOR results didn't accurately represent the research findings; rather, the published results used different time points when describing the gastrointestinal AE data, as well as the cardiac AEs data, than were reflected in the actual study. The result of highlighting only a subset of the total cardiac events was that the cardiac AE data looked better than it in fact was (Biddle 2007). Only years later were these publications called into question.

The above concerns were not the only ethical lapses in the VIGOR trial. Krumholz et al. point out that several prominent medical journals did not adequately employ peer review that might have caught some of the above issues; furthermore, once problems were found, the correction process on the part of journals wasn't entirely robust. At least one article that spoke favorably about Vioxx was ghost-written by consultants hired by Merck (Ross et al. 2008). There were many failures and lessons to be learned from rofecoxib, and it is of course easy with 20/20 hindsight to try to second-guess what may have happened. One takeaway is that independent and rigorous data safety monitoring is essential to clinical trials. "Independent data and safety monitoring boards should be mandated and their governance should not be under the control of the company" (Krumholtz et al. 2007, 122).

There is an interesting postscript to the Vioxx story. An additional study of rofecoxib to see if it could prevent colon polyps, the Adenomatous Polyp Prevention on Vioxx (APPROVe) study, was started in 2000. The APPROVe data safety monitoring committee halted that study after only eighteen months, after 3.5 percent of patients taking Vioxx experienced a heart attack, with only 1.9 percent of patients in a placebo arm experiencing that AE. The APPROVe study resulted in Vioxx being pulled off the market (Biddle 2007). APPROVe's DMC members were deposed as part of lawsuits brought by participants in the trial, although they were not defendants in the trial (DeMets and Ellenburg, 2016).

The VIGOR trial illustrates what is at stake in having unbiased, rigorous, and transparent monitoring. Rofecoxib was given to a large number of clinical trial participants even after it was found to raise cardiac risks, and then was permitted to be marketed to patients. There are many individuals tasked with protecting human participants and future cohorts of patients—the IRB, researchers, sponsors, medical monitors, and DSMBs. The VIGOR DSMB was one body in the monitoring process that could have prevented harm. The APPROVe DSMB stepped in with their own concerns, but by then, a great deal of damage had been done.

Conclusion

IRBs may be more familiar to bioethicists, but they are not the only committee tasked with ensuring that research participants are treated ethically.

DSMBs, with their unique history and charge, are an essential complement to the IRB system. While IRBs were created primarily to stop unethical research before it starts, DSMBs are charged with the ongoing oversight of research projects.

The reactive history of the IRB can be contrasted with the proactive history of the DSMB. DSMBs are fortunate in having a history that positions them not as regulating unscrupulous researchers but as collaborators in the research enterprise. DSMBs have a powerful role in shaping research, one that hasn't always claimed center stage. The importance of responsible data safety monitoring may only come to light in its absence.

However, despite the contributions of DSMBs, they have been less studied by bioethicists than IRBs. Perhaps the first question to answer is, What does the ethicist offer to DSMB deliberations? If the DSMB comprises specialists whose unique background allows them to evaluate a project in process, then what does the bioethicist bring to the table? How does the ethicist's unique insights contribute to keeping research participants safe? That is the topic of the next chapter.

2   What Does an Ethicist Bring to the DSMB?
The STRIVE-IPF Trial

Idiopathic pulmonary fibrosis (IPF) is a chronic lung disease. When the disease suddenly worsens (called an acute exacerbation), IPF can result in a swift decline in health. Patients who experience acute exacerbation of idiopathic pulmonary fibrosis (AE-IPF) may have only weeks or months to live. Although treating pulmonologists do their best to manage AE-IPF with steroids or antibiotics, there are no known curative treatments, or even widely successful maintenance therapies. The STRIVE-IPF (Study of Therapeutic Plasma Exchange, Rituximab and Intravenous Immunoglobulin for Acute Exacerbations of Idiopathic Pulmonary Fibrosis) trial was designed to test a new therapy for AE-IPF. Patients were randomized in a 2:1[1] ratio into either 1) an arm that included steroids, antibiotics, and therapeutic plasma exchange plus rituximab plus intravenous immunoglobulin or 2) treatment as usual (TAU), which included steroids and antibiotics.[2]

The Ethicist at the Table

DSMBs are assembled with specialist knowledge so as best to monitor the research studies they oversee. Unlike IRBs, which may review diverse projects and have Common Rule guidelines as to their membership, DSMB members are selected with expert backgrounds in the trials they monitor but have no uniform guidelines about membership. IRB's are site specific—a given hospital's IRB, for example, will review all research from principal investigators who work at that hospital. Thus, IRBs may review research across a wide variety of disciplines. DSMBs, by contrast, are project-specific—they are assembled on a case-by-case basis for individual projects. In some cases, DSMBs are convened to provide oversight for several projects in a single discipline, or of the same drug, but in distinct therapeutic areas. The size of a DSMB may be smaller or larger, depending on the complexity of the study and the potential risk of harm to participants. DSMBs typically include clinicians who are familiar with the condition under study, but without any conflicts of interest that might compromise their objectivity. Cardiology trials are overseen by cardiologists; infectious disease trials are overseen by infectious disease specialists. Ideally, these practitioners also have expertise in clinical trial methodology, although DeMets and Ellenberg (2016, 1370) caution, "The number of scientists who have experience with and training for DMC activity has not kept pace. As a result, many people are asked to serve on numerous DMCs; however, some DMCs are operating with less-experienced members." In addition to clinicians who specialize in medical aspects of the trial, most DSMBs have a biostatistician who specializes in design, management, and data collection in clinical trials. The expertise of these clinical and statistical specialists may be augmented by adding individuals to the DSMB who have additional specialized knowledge (for example, the DSMB for the CALEC Trial, discussed in chapter 3, included two experts in stem cell manufacture). Although not a member of the DSMB, closed sessions of DSMB meetings typically include an unblinded statistician not otherwise involved with the study who prepares interim reports and can offer additional insight into the protocol if needed (Gordon, Sugarman, and Kass 1998).

In addition to these specialists, many DSMBs have—or many should have, in my opinion, if they don't already—an ethicist who specializes in clinical research (Friedman and Schron 2008). Although this is my admittedly biased opinion, it isn't uniformly shared. The DAMOCLES study group found that "no consensus was reached about ethicist or consumer or lay membership" on data monitoring committees (DAMOCLES 2005, 712). The World Health Organization's "Operational Guidelines for the Establishment and Functioning of Data Safety Monitoring Boards" advocates including an ethicist, but not in all cases: membership "should include individuals with relevant clinical and statistical expertise. Additional expertise may be required in certain studies, e.g. in the specific disease area being studied, or in ethics" (2005, 10). The NIH's 1998 guidelines recommend that DSMB membership include "clinical trial experts, biostatisticians, bioethicists, and clinicians knowledgeable about the disease and treatment under study" (NIH 1998). The FDA's nonbinding recommendations state, "For trials with unusually high risks or with broad public health implications, the DMC may include a medical ethicist knowledgeable about the design, conduct, and interpretation of clinical trials" (U.S. Department of Health and Human

Services 2006, 8), and distinguish the role of an ethicist from a patient advocate: "someone with the disease or condition under study or a close relative of such an individual, for example" (8). Herson's recommendations are similar, noting that ethicists or patient advocates are typically "ad hoc consultants" who may have a routine role in NIH-sponsored trials, but are typically only engaged on monitoring committees in industry-sponsored trials if there are pressing ethical issues that are expected to emerge (Herson 2017, 26). The European Medicines Agency offers a tempered endorsement of ethicists on DMCs: "As ethical aspects are important especially in safety monitoring, the inclusion of a member with expertise in ethical questions might be appropriate" (EMA 2005, 6). Cairns, Hallstrom, and Held don't endorse having an ethicist on every data monitoring committee, although "it is highly desirable that an ethical consultant be available for a DSMC to call on when needed" (Cairns, Hallstrom, and Held 2001, 161). On a less sanguine note, Kerr and Rawat (2023, 12) maintain, "Some have advocated for ethicists or patient advocates to be represented on the DMC. In truth, their presence on DMCs is extremely rare in current DMCs, and their lack of participation does not seem to have been detrimental." There isn't uniform endorsement of ethicists serving on a DSMBs, and it may be unnecessary or prohibitive for every DSMB to have an ethicist. Given the diversity of recommendations, it is necessary to discuss what an ethicist might contribute to DSMB deliberations.

One of the challenges in discussing the role of ethicists on DSMBs is that the title "ethicist" is contested. Chidwick et al. (2010, 32, 34) refer to the hospital-based clinical ethicist as an "unregulated profession" that "did not generally have formal job descriptions." Further complicating matters, Chidwick et al. observe the hospital-based clinical ethicist may have any one of several terminal professional degrees, including an MD or JD. White, Jankowski, and Shelton (2014) argue that clinical ethicists who engage in ethics consultations should qualify as such via a written exam demonstrating knowledge of the American Society of Bioethics and Humanities (ASBH's) core knowledge competencies. Individuals can receive a certificate through the ASBH as a health care ethics consultant;[3] however, this certification is focused on clinical ethicists consults, not research ethics. Only a minority of ethicists have this certification, and numerous authors have disputed White, Jankowski, and Shelton's conclusion. Brown and McGee (2014) argue that in addition to theoretical knowledge and expertise about ethics, ethicists should adopt the methodologies and practices of empirical researchers in the social sciences so as to expand their impact on health care. However, not all ethicists engage in empirical research. There is no consensus about the qualifications for an ethicist. Clarity about the role of ethicists on DSMBs are vexed by the fact that what qualifies someone as an "ethicist" is disputed in ways that the qualifications for "biostatistician" or "clinician" are not.

Perhaps the best way to identify a qualified DSMB ethicist is operationally, by examining the roles an ethicist serves on the DSMB and seeing if the person is able to perform successfully. The ethicist can serve multiple roles: someone who is well versed in policy regarding clinical trials, a patient advocate, and a person who is well positioned to ask the right questions of the clinical and statistical specialists to ensure the protection of human participants. Each of these distinct roles illustrates the complexity of DSMB deliberations. Just as the DSMB serves to protect the interests of human participants in a variety of ways, the ethicist may serve in multiple roles.

The Ethicist as Policy Expert

Each DSMB ethicist should be an expert on the policies that guide ethical research. The ethicist comes to the table with a complete understanding of documents such as the *Belmont Report*, the Common Rule, and the Declaration of Helsinki. In some cases, DSMBs review research projects after they have been developed by principal investigators and their team and after the project has undergone an initial review by the IRB of record. In this capacity, the DSMB communicates to the researchers, the sponsor, and the IRB, recommending final edits on a consent document or recruitment materials, as well as on the methodology, data collection strategy, statistical analysis plans (including data shells that reflect which data and how those data will be reported to the DSMB), AE reporting, and monitoring plan. In my experience, serving as a DSMB member for NIH-sponsored projects, the development of consent documents is often an iterative process in which the DSMB examines a consent document vetted by the IRB of record, the DSMB offers suggestions, and the IRB then has the final word on those recommendations.

In my role as the ethics policy expert on DSMBs, I have been charged with a thorough review of informed consent documents. The expectation is that the ethicist knows all the requirements of informed consent documents per the Common Rule, such as clear statements that participation is voluntary; the risks, benefits, alternatives, and the costs of research; confidentiality protections; the number of participants in the trial and number of sites from which they will be recruited; and contact information so the participants can reach out with questions or execute a responsible withdrawal from the study (45 CFR §46.117). Consent documents need to include all the above information, written so that prospective participants can understand and make an informed decision to participate based on that understanding. Since ethicists aren't experts in the clinical aspects of the research, but are still conversant in the study's methodology, they are positioned to translate complex clinical language into language better suited to potential participants. I've worked closely with research teams to formulate novel ways to make consent documents shorter, to add white space, or to describe medical procedures using analogies drawn from everyday experience. For example, in the STRIVE-IPF study, I assisted in shortening the informed consent document, recommending a presentation of various tests and procedures on the consent form to promote clarity without repetitiveness.[4]

The role of policy expert is perhaps the most straightforward role of the DSMB ethicist. Just as the clinicians or statisticians on the DSMB come to the table with clinical or statistical expertise, the ethicist comes to the table with ethics expertise: expertise in codes of conduct, expertise in the application of ethical theories and principles, and expertise in the history of research ethics that may prevent researchers from repeating the mistakes of the past. In the role of policy expert, the ethicist may be most helpful to DSMBs overseeing trials in which participants' safety is most at risk because there are significant unknowns about the risks of the trial, because the therapies under study are known to carry significant risks, or because the size or complexity of the trial may contribute to the likelihood of risk to participants.

The Ethicist as Patient Advocate

Beyond ethical expertise, the DSMB ethicist is often cast in the role of patient advocate. As stated in chapter 1, DSMB guidelines are not uniform, which extends to claims about DSMB membership. For example, The National Cancer Institute (NCI) of the NIH says in its "Policy of The National Cancer Institute for Data and Safety Monitoring of Clinical Trials" that DSMB membership should include "lay representatives selected based on their experience, reputation for objectivity, absence of conflicts of interest (and the appearance of same), and knowledge of clinical trial methodology" (National Cancer Institute NCI Clinical and Translational Research Operations Committee 2014), whereas the National Eye Institute only states that the DSMC (their preferred terminology) should include "public representatives" (National Eye Institute 2021). These "lay" or "public" representatives are often individuals who have firsthand experience as either patients or caregivers of patients with the condition under study. Calis et al., in a survey and focus group study of data monitoring committees, observed that patient advocates are useful "especially for trials including patient-reported outcomes, quality-of-life measures, or a comparative effectiveness research design" (2017, 62). Notably, focus group participants drew a distinction between patient advocates and ethicists. In some cases, patient representatives are well-known public advocates for services and funding, and in others, they are not the public face of the condition, but individuals who are meant to represent the daily experience of a typical patient or caregiver.

The ethicist serving on the DSMB may not have the firsthand experience of the patient advocate but may be pressed into the role of advocating for patients, in addition to the role of ethicist. There are two sides to this dual casting of the ethicist, but it is important to recognize that ethicists assuming the role of patient advocate isn't unmitigated good news.

One positive aspect of the patient advocate role includes the recognition that patients *do* need an advocate, and the ethicist is at the table, in part, to fulfill that role. Historically, patients and potential research participants haven't had a voice in the development and oversight of clinical research. The NCI's recommendation, above, goes some distance to remedying this oversight.

The DSMB's ethicist as patient advocate may be a cousin to the community representative on the IRB. The Common Rule requires that all IRBs have at least five members, one of whom is a "scientific" professional, one of whom is a "nonscientific" member. and at least one "non-affiliated" member (45 CFR §46.107(b)–(c)). This "non-affiliated" member is often referred to as a "community representative." Dresser maintains that the role of "outsiders" in ethical oversight emerged from the assumption that physicians and scientists would place their interests in the trials above the interests of research participants (Dresser 2008, 232). Installing nonscientific and community members on IRBs creates a counterbalance to those whose interests aren't sufficiently focused on participants. Since the nonscientific member and the community member can be the same individual, often a single person occupies both roles (Klitzman 2015). What distinguishes the IRB's "non-affiliated member" isn't defined, except in a negative sense: "Each IRB shall include at least one member who is not otherwise affiliated with the institution and who is not part of the immediate family of a person who is affiliated with the institution" (45 CFR §46.07(c)). Beyond this negative claim about what the community member *isn't*, little is said about who the community member *is*. Is the community member part of the *geographic* community in which the research is taking place, or a member of the *community of illness* from which the participant population will be drawn? This is left open to (mis)interpretation. Klitzman catalogues several studies in which community members often feel unheard and not respected among their IRB colleagues (Klitzman 2015, 49–50). Merely being a member of the general public, without a stake in the research at hand, doesn't guarantee that the community representative will advocate, or be an effective advocate, on the part of potential participants (Dresser 2017, 3). Community members may even be seen as being co-opted by the researchers with whom they work (Dresser 2008, 234). More troubling is the fact that the IRB "community member" has second-class status: IRBs are permitted to convene and vote on protocols when their non-affiliated member isn't present (45 CFR §46.108(b)).

One way in which the DSMB ethicist is distinct from the IRB "community representative" harkens back to the unique role of the DSMB, in contrast to the IRB. As pointed out above, IRBs are "site specific," reviewing multiple projects that may range across diverse areas of specialization, whereas DSMBs are convened with specific projects in mind. As such, the DSMB's ethicist is chosen to complement the clinical and statistical expertise of other DSMB members. The ethicist isn't chosen by virtue of what they *aren't*; rather, they are chosen because of their expertise in clinical trials. Some community members on IRBs are chosen by happenstance, convenience, or word-of-mouth among informal networks, not necessarily because they are representative of the "community" (Klitzman 2015, 50).

Ideally, the ethicist on the DSMB is able to act as a patient advocate because they are sufficiently well versed in the study's clinical and statistical methodology so as to be able to speak to concerns patients may have. For example, in the SIGHT study discussed in chapter 5, participants underwent a Humphrey visual field test. The Humphrey visual field test measures an individual's range of vision (how many degrees a person can see side to side, left to right, right to left, and up and down without moving their head). According to investigators, patients didn't like this test at all, even though it played a significant role in the study. It wasn't an option to eliminate the Humphrey visual field test; at the same time, its inclusion also presented a risk of harm to participants.[5] Since I had never experienced a Humphrey visual field test, I asked a technician who wasn't involved in the research why it was so stressful. Was the test onerous? Was it painful? Did it require special preparation? The answer was none of the above. Instead, many patients often felt "judged" when they took the test, believing they "failed" if they were unable to answer the questions, causing anxiety.[6] This understanding allowed me to better advocate for patients undergoing the procedure as part of data collection. Although I had never taken a Humphrey visual field test, it was within my power to learn more so that the participants I represented had a voice at the table.

My lack of clinical background allows me to read informed consent documents from the perspective of a patient, not glossing over technical terms or vague descriptions of medical procedures owing to clinical familiarity. Klitzman observes a similar advantage holds true for some community IRB members who "may play a particularly unique and important role by reviewing consent forms, in part because physician members recognize that they themselves have difficulty reading these documents as a lay-person would" (Klitzman 2015, 54). This outsider perspective allows an ethicist to identify questions or concerns research participants might have. To present a mundane example, I recall a consent form I reviewed, which stated that as part of the data collection, "two fecal samples" would be analyzed. I requested clarification: Did patients have to give two samples, or would they only have to give a single sample, which would be analyzed twice? Because participants are *definitely going to prefer* the latter over the former, make no mistake; thus, they should be adequately informed as to what was being asked of them. It may be obvious to clinicians—"*two samples* means we'll be asking for two, twice, two times"—but for the patient, this may not be obvious at all.

By virtue of not being a clinician, the ethicist's imaginative empathy allows them to see the protocol from the standpoint of the research participant. When I'm sitting in a room with several clinicians discussing the process of undergoing a tedious, difficult, or painful procedure, I don't picture myself as the treating clinician. I don't have the background, training, or practice to immediately see myself in that role. Instead, I picture myself as the participant. I empathize with what that participant is going through and the questions that might run through their head: How long is this going to take? Will it hurt? I had to fast for the last eighteen hours before this test—when will I get to eat? Training as an ethicist imbues me with historical and policy background, and my *lack* of clinical background provides me with a perspective that is participant oriented. In this way, the DSMB ethicist is akin to some conceptions of the IRB community member whose role is to empathize with the participant rather than the researchers.

One negative aspect of the "patient advocate" role is that training as an ethicist doesn't afford anyone with special knowledge about patient advocacy (Persad 2014). Ethicists know the unique history of exploitation of research participants and policies in place to protect participants, but that doesn't guarantee that the ethicist will be an effective advocate if such exploitation looms again. Being an ethicist isn't the same as being a strong advocate. But it does give one a framework to consider research from an ethical, not clinical, perspective.

Some may point to this empathetic reasoning behind the role of the patient advocate as limited. If it is best for members of a given group to be at the table to advocate for members of that group, the ethicist may be at a loss when they are not members of that group. This is a problem—although I can research the experience of undergoing a Humphrey visual field test, I don't know what it is like to be a man undergoing a prostate exam or to be a Black woman being evaluated for prenatal hypertension. Imaginative empathy places me in the place of the participant rather than the clinician, but there are constraints as to how far imaginative empathy can take me. I do my best to always be thinking of the participants' perspective, while at the same time realizing my limits.

Dresser argues for more extensive engagement with patients who are experiencing the diseases under study in ethics committees, precisely because those firsthand experiences cannot be replicated. The patient perspective has often been shortchanged. Having a patient advocate who is actually a patient—in addition to an ethicist—on DSMBs would only expand the DSMB's understanding (Dresser 2017, 270). A somewhat dissenting opinion comes from Rand Rosenblatt: "Rand Rosenblatt worries that a participant representative might provide a veneer of approval without substantively influencing the board's decisions" (Persad 2014, 159, referencing Rosenblatt 1978). This is a realistic concern. Claiming that there is a patient advocate on any board—whether a grant review panel, an IRB, or a DSMB—may mask genuine dissent on the part of that advocate. In the worst case, the patient advocate serving as a member gives the patina of legitimacy to a board's decisions, even those antithetical to what patients or their advocates would want. Having a patient advocate on the DSMB is only as successful as other members' willingness to take that individual seriously. Given the hierarchical nature of medicine in the United States, it is occasionally a challenge for my perspective to be taken seriously by some DSMB members. A fortiori, a "lay" patient or advocate may be even more encumbered. This is not an argument against lay membership on DSMBs; it is a call for all DSMB members to take seriously the concerns of each member, regardless of their background.

Persad cites a related concern: Including patient advocates on IRBs, for example, would "overbureaucratize" those boards, as IRBs might opt for representation from "advocates" rather than participants themselves (Persad 2014, 163). It is true that not all advocates are ideal representatives; not all participants' concerns will necessarily be voiced by those chosen to represent the whole of the participant experience. Dresser dubs this the "heterogeneity problem"—the fact that each participant's experiences are unique, and hence, no one participant can be expected to stand in for the multiplicity of patient experiences (Dresser 2017, 282). Ultimately, however, Rosenblatt and Persad endorse greater participation from individuals such as research participants on boards that decide their cohort's fate, not merely as a means of securing certain outcomes but as a way of exercising the right to be heard in democratic deliberations.

The concerns raised above about equating the ethicist with patient advocate revolve around the possibility that equating their roles might shortchange patient advocacy. The flip side of that coin is that equating the ethicist with patient advocate diminishes the specialized knowledge *the ethicist* brings to the table. If all that an ethicist contributes is the empathetic connection with participants—speaking up on their behalf—then why have someone with specialist training as an ethicist on the DSMB? Wouldn't any patient advocate, such as a current or former patient with the condition under study, serve just as well? This position is mistaken, in my estimation, because some aspects of protecting human participants *do* require specialized knowledge. When and how a legally authorized representative (LAR) can consent for a participant, the distinction between a LAR's decision being based on a substituted judgment or a best-interest standard, and what that means for the protection of patient autonomy are not lay knowledge. Professional ethicists are able to share expert understanding about Common Rule requirements for informed consent, the distinctions between assent and consent, and the types of protection afforded by a Certificate of Confidentiality, to name but a few. Just as clinicians on a DSMB bring specialized clinical knowledge, and statisticians bring specialized statistical knowledge, the ethicist brings formalized training in ethical protections and policy issues. It is the ethicist's role to impart their specialized knowledge to the members of the DSMB, so that together they can collaborate on the protection of human participants.

Ultimately, I have come to appreciate my dual role. Merely being *named* as "ethicist and patient advocate" helps to remind me of my function on the DSMB. I am there to advocate for participants—it is part of my title. Rather than view that status as a diminution of my role as someone with specialized ethical training, I chose to embrace the dual role of ethics expert *and* the sole individual on the DSMB whose titled responsibility is to speak on behalf of participants.

There are many situations in which it would be ideal to have DSMB membership that includes *both* an ethicist and patient advocate, each serving in distinct roles on the board. In that way, the DSMB's expertise would expand to incorporate both ethical reasoning as well as a first-person patient-oriented perspective. Their expertise would be welcome and would complement the clinical, statistical, and ethical expertise already reflected on many DSMBs. Dresser points out, however, that including a patient advocate on ethics committees doesn't solve the "heterogeneity problem." Each patient advocate may end up speaking for themselves, not the diverse concerns of other potential participants. Thus, even incorporating a prior or current participant on each DSMB isn't a perfect solution. As it stands, there are many cases in which the ethicist on the DSMB is expected to take on the role of both ethicist and patient advocate. But for the ethicist at the DSMB table, the contributions don't end there.

Bringing an Ethicist's Perspective

In addition to policy expertise and serving as a patient advocate, the ethicist brings a perspective to DSMB discussions beyond that had by clinicians and statisticians. The ethicist can raise questions about the clinical, methodological, or statistical parameters of a trial, which can inspire other experts on the DSMB to revise their thinking. For this reason, the ethicist should be conversant in some clinical aspects of the trial as well as statistical boundaries and guidelines that inform the trial. When trials potentially place subjects at higher risks (a topic discussed in chapter 3) or approach the boundary of falling out of equipoise or futility (discussed in chapter 4), an ethicist needs to engage clinicians and statisticians on the ethical issues that emerge.

The ethicist is often able to see data in a new light, owing to their formalized training in ethics and policy. This is slightly different from the former claim about imaginative empathy—allowing me to place myself in the position of a participant when reading a consent form, or undergoing study exams. Rather, the ethicist on the DSMB, being an outsider among the clinical and statistical specialists, creates opportunities to examine scientific findings presented to the DSMB from a nonscientific perspective. That was the case in the NHLBI-sponsored STRIVE-IPF trial.

Patients with AE-IPF typically don't live very long because the disease is so damaging and treatment options are so limited. The primary endpoint—the leading result that the researchers were attempting to achieve with the experimental treatment—was six-month survival beyond the date participants were randomized into the study. The enormity of that primary endpoint cannot be stressed enough: The experimental therapy would be considered successful if the proportion of participants who lived at least six months after randomization was statistically higher than the proportion of control. The participants and evaluators were "blinded" as to which arm participants occupied—either the TAU arm or the rituximab and intravenous immunoglobulin arm. Some members of the research team who prepared the infusions knew which participants were receiving the experimental infusions and which were receiving TAU. But the assessment of the patients' progress was collected by different individuals from those who administered the experimental infusions, which is to say that the assessment of participant progress was done in a double-blind manner. The study began in fall of 2018 and was initially scheduled through summer 2022,[7] with the DSMB meeting every six months. Both the efficacy data (about how well patients were doing) and the AE data (which tracked the frequency and magnitude of harmful side effects) were reported in those meetings, in aggregate form.[8] Prior to the study commencing, the DSMB had agreed on the type of data they wanted to see and how the data were to be reported. Typically, the data shells—tables or charts that are used to present data, including a discussion of what data are relevant for the DSMB to review—are agreed to by the DSMB before a study commences. These data shells are then populated with the study data as the trial progresses and may be subject to change as data emerge that impact the safety and outcome of the trial.

Everything was going according to plan as the first few DSMB meetings took place. As patients enrolled across the multiple sites, there were no safety signals in either arm that indicated the study should be altered in any way. Although the discussions of pulmonary medicine, or the statistics behind the complex trial, were not in my wheelhouse, I attended every meeting and followed along with the conversation. Data as to how long patients were living, which showed the possible benefits of the trial, and data on AEs, which showed the risks of harm from the trial, were being aggregated in different groups, per the previously agreed-upon data shells. The Department of Health and Human Services defines *adverse events* as "any untoward or unfavorable medical occurrence in a human subject, including any abnormal sign (for example, abnormal physical exam or laboratory finding), symptom, or disease, temporally associated with the subject's participation in the research, whether or not considered related to the subject's participation in the research."[9] SAEs are those that result in death, are life-threatening, require in-patient hospital treatment, or result in disability or a birth defect. However, there were no individualized data tracking which individual participants were experiencing which AEs. As the study progressed, one question nagged at me: *What if the patients who were living longer were living longer with increasingly more bad side effects?*

A short aside on a controversy that occasionally arises on DSMBs: In some trials the DSMB is intentionally blinded to study arms. Demographic, efficacy, AE, and enrollment data are reported, but the DSMB is not told which study arms are which. The assumption is that just as researchers and participants are not informed about which patients occupy which study arms, so as to reduce bias, so too should DSMBs be kept blinded about study arm data so as to reduce bias. Keeping DSMBs blinded to the study arms is considered by many a controversial choice, with Curtis Meinert going so far as to call it "blind stupidity" (Meinert 1998; see also Department of Health and Human Services Office of the Inspector General 2013; U.S. Department of Health and Human Services 2006, 14; Wakim and Shaw 2018, 137–138). Per the DAMOCLES study group, "blinding is generally not recommended for DMC members, although opinions vary" (DAMOCLES 2005, 719). Herson assesses what committees should do if they are masked to treatment assignments, advocating a decision matrix that allows committee members to project what they would do if they were unmasked, so as to inform a choice to remain masked or not (Herson 2017, 140). Whether or not the data are presented in a way that allows the DSMB to uphold its mission of keeping participants safe is itself an ethical question. DeMets and Freidman recount the experience of the Cardiac Arrhythmia Suppression Trial (CAST), which like the STRIVE-IPF trial, was sponsored by the NHLBI (DeMets and Friedman 2006). CAST was a placebo-controlled randomized controlled trial (RCT) initially designed to examine three drugs—encainide, flecainide, and moriezine—on 4,400 patients with ventricular arrhythmias and reduced ventricular function. After a run-in period to examine if participants responded to any of the drugs, the study commenced, with the primary endpoint being death from arrhythmia. CAST's DSMB initially "decided to remain partially blinded in their review of interim data" (DeMets and Friedman 2006, 202), a decision they were forced to reverse after detecting a high incidence of the primary endpoint in some arms. Unblinding demonstrated the endpoint was higher in the encainide and flecainide arms than in others. Those arms were discontinued, leaving the moricizie and placebo arms. However, a subsequent increase in deaths during the run-in period required unblinding of the data yet again, which showed that the moricizine arm experienced higher deaths. The DSMB met one more time and, upon seeing a further increase in deaths of participants taking moricizine in the run-in period, recommended the study be halted. The CAST experience can serve as a cautionary tale about the harms to participants when DSMBs are blinded to study arms. If a sponsor is unwilling to share data DSMB members believe they need in order to keep participants safe, the DSMB members may wish to rethink their involvement in monitoring the study.

Questions of blinding the DSMB were not an issue in the STRIVE-IPF trial—the concern was *not* that the DSMB was intentionally prevented from receiving data that could inform their assessment of the study. Rather, patient-level data that could inform the DSMB whether patients were living longer only to experience more AEs were not reported. The aggregate data were available, but aggregate data may be misleading. AEs can "cluster" around individual participants and, at particular time-points for each participant—the patient who experiences an SAE that requires hospitalization may not experience the precipitating SAE in isolation. Instead, a flood of AEs may surround the precipitating SAE. In the absence of patient-level data tracking AEs over time, it was difficult to parse if participants were living longer, only to experience more AEs.

Even if participants were living longer only to experience more AEs, that might not have been reason to stop the study. For one, patients with acute exacerbations of IPF are very sick. If those receiving the experimental treatment were living longer, they were probably also experiencing more AEs simply by virtue of living longer. Sick people who live longer are sicker for longer. But in addition to that fact, it may be the case that for some patients, experiencing SAEs, such as frequent hospitalization, was an acceptable trade-off in exchange for living a few more weeks, or months, of life. Imagine an IPF patient who wanted to live long enough to see a child's wedding or a grandchild's graduation. For that patient, a few more months of life, even punctuated with SAEs, may be worth it. Other patients may choose quality of life rather than living a few extra months. Patients have autonomy rights to make decisions about what they believe is in their best interest. Physicians should not paternalistically assume their own notion of beneficence is the last word in what is in the best interests of their patients. As such, collecting data as to whether or not patients were living longer, but were doing so while experiencing a greater number of AEs, wasn't tantamount to demonstrating that the study was unsuccessful. Rather, it was another piece in the puzzle that would help inform researchers what the data meant.

Asking questions about the trade-off between quality of life and quantity of life is familiar territory for bioethicists. Tom Beauchamp and James F. Childress (2019), for example, in their discussion of the principle of beneficence, examine the complexities in using cost-effectiveness analysis, cost-benefit analysis, and the value of quality adjusted-life years (QALYs) as measures of successful treatments. A well-used metric, QALYs are a means of measuring the health outcome of a course of treatment based upon "the length and quality of life" (Beauchamp and Childress 2019, 254, quoting National Institute for Health and Clinical Excellence). For example, in determining if it is better to maintain an elderly terminal emphysema patient on a hospital's last ventilator or to attempt to reallocate the ventilator to a far younger patient with what may be a transient case of pneumonia, one may use QALYs to determine which patient is expected to have more high-quality years of life ahead of them. QALYs may be used in both treatment and research frameworks (Beauchamp and Childress 2019, 254). Beauchamp and Childress rightly point out that the use of QALYs to guide treatment decisions is predicated on ethical assumptions, such as the claim that health maximization is the only value worth protecting in medicine; or that QALYs may discriminate against older people, racial minorities, and the disabled by placing greater value on the life years of the younger and able-bodied; or that the use of QALYs is too utilitarian, such that other ethical imperatives, like a duty of rescue, are diminished in the face of maximizing QALYs (Beauchamp and Childress 2019, 255–256). Riviello et al. (2022) analyzed preemptive scoring of 498 intensive care patients using a "crisis standards of care" system, designed to maximize numbers-of-life years, in one Boston hospital during a COVID-19 surge. They found "nearly twice the proportion of Black patients were scored in the lowest priority group compared with all other patients" (Riviello et al. 2022, 1). A focus on quality-of-life years, as demonstrated by Riviello et al., can significantly bias decision-making. Similarly, disability studies scholars have pushed back against the use of QALYs, instead embracing metrics such as "full quality of life," given each individual's unique circumstances (Franklin 2017) or respecting reasonable patient preferences (Davies 2019).

Another area of bioethics in which the trade-off between quality of life and length of life is extensively discussed is end-of-life decision-making. Ezekiel Emanuel has publicly stated that he doesn't want any life-extending treatments after the age of seventy-five because the expected decline in quality of life would render him, and the way that he is remembered by others, diminished (Emanuel 2014). A narrative approach to these questions urges end-of-life decision-making on the part of surrogates to be consistent with the life story of the patient (Lo 2023). Some end-of-life conversations are about whether a patient wants, or would want, to extend life despite a perceived diminishment in quality of life. There is no one-size-fits-all answer to this question—each patient, or patient's surrogates, should have the right to make that decision themselves. It isn't for the DSMB to make a value judgment whether a given course of treatment is preferable for one participant over the other—that would be just as paternalistic as the treating physician making the decision for a patient.

However, knowing that one arm of the STRIVE-IPF study bought patients longer lives, but at the price of a greater number of AEs or SAEs, would be an important result of the study. If therapeutic plasma exchange plus rituximab plus intravenous immunoglobulin was approved for patient use and resulted in longer life even with more side effects, patients would need to know this before electing that course of treatment. They could then make an informed choice based on their values and preferences. If, however, the patients who were living longer were *also* living with fewer AEs or SAEs—that would be unambiguously good news. As the STRIVE-IPF DSMB looked at the aggregate data, there was no way to tell if the participants who were living longer were also living better. The copious data tables provided by the study's own statisticians weren't enough to answer my question. It was clear that a new way of looking at the data would need to be conceived to find an answer.

My question prompted a way of presenting the trial data beyond that in the preapproved data shells. A collaborative suggestion emerged for a visual representation of the data that would address my concern: a timeline for each patient that represented their trajectory, including SAEs such as a hospitalization and nonserious AEs. Previously unbeknownst to me, this is referred to as a *swim lane* map or diagram, also referred to as a *process flow diagram*. Swim lane diagrams are akin to a flowchart in which each individual participant is given their own lane to map their progress in the study (Minnesota Department of Public Health 2023). Each participant's individual trajectory is presented along a timeline, marked by symbols to represent AEs and SAEs. The swim lanes would allow the DSMB to discern whether patients were living longer only to experience more AEs and SAEs, or whether living longer was also correlated with comparatively high quality of life.

My role as an ethicist, asking a very typical ethicist question about quality of life, contributed to the DSMB's deeper understanding of the experiences of the participants in the STRIVE-IPF trial. Preapproved data shells aren't the limit of what a DSMB is expected to know about a trial. When additional data are needed to have a complete picture of what is happening, the DSMB has the authority, the right, and the responsibility to ask for those data.[10] As discussed above, if the DSMB believes that being blinded to the arms of the study will compromise their ability to do their job, they should demand a presentation of the data consistent with their mission. The dynamic nature of clinical trials means responsible DSMBs should exercise their authority to ask for more data, or additional presentations of those data, if additional information is required to protect participants. Knowing in each individual participant's case if life was being prolonged, only for it to be of lower quality, was fundamental to understanding if STRIVE-IPF was a success. This type of contribution is one of the most significant that an ethicist can make—allowing the other members of the DSMB to look at data in new ways so that participants can be better protected throughout the trial. The ethicist doesn't have to be the gadfly, pushing against the judgment of the clinicians and statisticians. Rather, the ethicist can urge novel ways of looking at existing data—ways that promote better research.

Conclusion

There is no uniform agreement that an ethicist is required on each DSMB, but there are compelling ways an ethicist can improve DSMB deliberations, especially in studies in which there is a greater risk of potential harm to participants or there are significant unknowns that can jeopardize the safety of participants. One of the contributions of an ethicist on a DSMB is to bring an outside perspective to deliberations. The ethicist is an expert in the ethical execution of human research, applying the Common Rule as well as other policies to contribute to participant safety. The ethicist is also often cast in the role of a patient advocate, although that role can be a vexed one. The role of patient advocate may assume too much expertise on the part of ethicists, in terms of understanding what participants may experience in the trial as well as a presumption of expertise as an advocate. There may be some cases in which an additional DSMB member who is a current or former patient may better take up that mantel. I see my role as both ethicist and patient advocate as an honor, reminding me that patients are counting on me to be their voice.

In addition to these important roles, the ethicist on the DSMB can find ways to cast the study data in a new light, as illustrated by the STRIVE-IPF trial. The ethicist on the DSMB, in asking questions that might not initially occur to statisticians or clinicians, can contribute to keeping human participants safe from undue risks of research. The ethicist is someone whose bioethics training allows them to ask challenging questions, in some cases creating opportunities for other members of the DSMB to bring their expertise to bear in new ways.

3 Measuring Risks, Informing Participants: The CALEC Trial

Limbal cells grow along the barrier between the eye's cornea and the conjunctiva (a barrier that covers the white part of the eye). Without healthy limbal cells, the conjunctiva can grow over the cornea, impairing vision. Limbal cell deficiency can be the result of traumatic eye injury, such as chemical or thermal burns. If a person's limbal cells are damaged in one eye, it may be possible to transplant healthy limbal cells from their undamaged eye to the damaged eye, thereby preventing the visual impairment from unimpeded growth of the conjunctiva. The standard of care in the United States for this type of transplant is CLAU, conjunctival-limbal autograft. One of the drawbacks of CLAU is that it requires a fair amount of limbal cells from the healthy eye to repair the damaged eye. Might a new procedure—CALEC transplantation—be better? CALEC takes far fewer limbal stem cells from the healthy eye than are used in CLAU and then uses a technique to grow those stem cells in a laboratory. A sheet of limbal cells is then available to transplant into the healthy eye. The CALEC study began as an investigation to compare the success of CALEC vs. CLAU.[1]

Step One: Weighing Risks against Benefits before a Study Begins

All research on human beings proceeds from the assumption that ethical research results in greater possible benefits than risks. It would be unethical to commence a research project knowing the benefits of the research would be outweighed by the risks. The benefits, such as possible benefits of new therapies as well as increased knowledge, may be experienced by participants but are more likely to fall to *future cohorts of patients* who in many cases have the same condition as the one under study. Research participants may be randomized to an arm of the study that is ultimately not as successful as the other arm. They may be exposed to AEs which aren't adequately addressed initially because researchers didn't anticipate those AEs or SAEs. Research participants may be exposed to tests, both those with minimal risk and those that exceed minimal risk, so as to gain information about the safety of the intervention. The risks of research, including AEs and psychological stressors, as well as investments of time, are invariably borne by the research participants themselves. Since the potential risks of the study fall solely on the participants, but the majority of benefits are expected to fall on *future patients*, those potential risks to participants need to be carefully assessed. When a DSMB is named before participant accrual, a thorough and systemic measure of risk may be one of their first tasks. Since DSMBs are usually project-specific, their members are uniquely qualified to assess the potential risks and benefits of an experimental treatment. Their assessment carries special weight, owing to their expertise in the area under study. In cases in which a DSMB is asked for its recommendation before a trial commences, the potential risks of the trial need to be adequately calculated, with potential benefits expected to outweigh possible risks.

The risks of the CALEC study were fascinating to think about. Both CLAU and CALEC involved surgical procedures, retrieving cells from the healthy eye and transplanting them to the damaged eye. Possible risks of CALEC, for example, included the risks of anesthesia, the risks of harvesting the limbal stem cells, the risks of the surgical graft of the cultivated stem cells, and the risks of the failure of any of the above. These risks were familiar to the clinicians on the DSMB. There are risks that the autologous stem cells might not grow at the lab or might not grow into a sheet large enough to serve as a suitable graft. Thus, the participants might get halfway through a weeks-long procedure—first undergoing a successful surgery to harvest limbal stem cells, then waiting for the stem cells to generate—before learning the second surgery to graft the new limbal cells might never happen. The CALEC study was primarily a feasibility study to assess if CALEC was successful often enough to be adopted as an alternative to CLAU. As such, the primary endpoint wasn't that participant's vision would be better in their damaged eye; rather, the primary endpoint was that the limbal stem cell transplant was successful. However, even though better vision wasn't the primary endpoint, patients knew, and hoped, that enrolling in the study was the first step toward possibly recovering vision in their damaged eye. As such, the risk of a failure of the stem cells to grow in the lab, thereby thwarting a successful transplant, wasn't a *physical* risk to participants. Nevertheless, for those who were hoping that the transplant might restore some vision lost in their damaged eye, this setback could be psychologically harmful.

The DSMB needed to be mindful of these potential psychological risks, as well as the risks to employability or the risks of loss of time, while these two surgeries and multiple follow-up visits occurred. Each test, appointment, blood draw, or survey represents a data point to investigators, but also a burden to participants. It isn't enough in ethical research that the benefits outweigh the risks, but also that the risks of the research are minimized as much as possible. This means not exposing participants to additional interventions beyond those necessary to collect the data required. Each of these risks needs to be carefully weighed by the DSMB.

One of the complexities in initially randomizing some participants to CLAU, and some to CALEC, is that the CLAU procedure uses a larger number of limbal cells from the healthy eye to transplant into the damaged eye. With CALEC, since fewer cells are taken initially, as the basis for a larger sheet of cells is grown in a lab, *in principle* the risks of the CALEC surgery may be fewer. A second, more significant difference is that the CALEC procedure can be performed a second time if the sheet of stem cells doesn't grow or if the transplant is unsuccessful, owing to fewer limbal cells being taking in the first CALEC surgery. There are typically only enough limbal cells in a donor eye to perform CLAU once. Thus, the risks of the standard-of-care arm of the study (CLAU) may have been greater than the risks of the experimental arm. These differences might have caused someone pause, leading to a possible conclusion that the study was unethical from the start since the participants who were randomized to CLAU were facing surgery with a greater potential for harm than CALEC (a detailed discussion about weighing off the harms across different arms is considered in chapter 4). However, in the absence of evidence to demonstrate if the risks of CLAU really exceeded those of CALEC, this was mere speculation. Determining if CALEC resulted in a lower probability of risks to patients than CLAU is why the study was conducted in the first place.

There is a further aspect in which the CALEC study was unique. Imagine a study in which a damaged left eye received an injection, or a left eye with a cataract received an experimental new lens. In both cases, the presumption is that the risks would be to the left eye. If the eye that was damaged is the left eye, and the experimental treatment was on the left eye, it stands to reason that the risks would be primarily to the *left eye*. But in both the CLAU and the CALEC arms, the primary risks were not to the damaged eye, but instead to the *healthy donor eye* from which the limbal cells would be taken. This counterintuitive realization, that the eye receiving treatment of a limbal cell transplant was not the eye that bore the greatest risk of harm, transforms the understanding of the balance of potential benefits over risks. The damaged eye in the CALEC study, tragically, was already damaged. The healthy eye—the donor eye—was fine. But retrieving limbal cells from the healthy eye so as to transfer them to the damaged eye, or to grow enough limbal cells so as to have an adequate graft, put the participant's *one remaining healthy eye at potential risk*. The risk was very small but existed nonetheless. Every candidate for either CLAU or CALEC had one eye that was significantly damaged and a remaining healthy eye. Even a miniscule risk of harm to the healthy eye could have had life-altering repercussions. The difference between life with a single healthy eye and no healthy eye is immeasurable. As one clinician on the DSMB said, once a patient has a damaged eye, "They don't want you anywhere near their other eye."[2]

Recognizing that the primary risk of the study was a potential risk to the healthy eye is obvious, as spelled out here, but is nonetheless counterintuitive. The reflexive conclusion is to assume that the risks to the participant are risks the participant faces in light of needing to be in the study in the first place. If the left eye's vision is the one that is compromised and the treatment targets the left eye, then the primary risks are to the left eye. But in this case, the DSMB had to move beyond that reflexive conclusion, recognizing that the risks to the donor eye were the ones that were most significant. The lesson here is that DSMBs need to be imaginative and flexible when assessing the risks to participants. The risks of a study may not always seem obvious; it is the task of the DSMB to explore the study from every angle. Physical, psychological, and social risks all need to be taken into account. The potential risks of a study aren't always apparent. Having a DSMB with members who bring different perspectives to a study helps to clarify precisely what those risks are and whether the potential risks are outweighed by potential benefits.

Measuring risks may be more of an art than a science, in part because there is an inherent subjectivity in the amount of risk individuals are willing to bear. Alex John London proposed the following definition of "reasonable risk" in research: "Risks to individual research participants are reasonable just in case they (1) require the least amount of intrusion into the interests of participants that is necessary in order to facilitate sound scientific inquiry and (2) are consistent with an equal regard for the basic interests of study participants and the members of the larger community whose interests that research is intended to serve" (London 2007a, 591). The first claim is consistent with the Common Rule requirement that the potential risks are to be minimized as much as possible consistent with the data collection necessary to obtain generalizable data. The second claim appears to be a claim about justice and fairness in distribution of research risks to participants, ensuring that they do not bear risks that are disproportionate to the benefit of the generalized knowledge to themselves and cohorts of patients whom that knowledge may serve.

Rid, Emanuel, and Wendler undertook an empirical study in an attempt to develop "a systematic framework for evaluating the risks of research interventions" (2010, 1472). They named their method "systematic evaluation of research risks," or SEER, which compares the risks of research activities such as allergy skin testing or a liver biopsy with those of comparator daily activities and experiences, such as common colds or bone fractures. Rid, Emanuel, and Wendler enlisted four physicians, one nurse, and one philosopher to assess the magnitude of harm of different activities and used independent data to assess the probability of harm so that the appropriate comparator activities could be matched to research activities. Their empirical study may be an attempt to quantify what London believes is one of the "operational criteria" for responsible research: "Identify social activities that are structurally similar to the research enterprise and (to) ensure that the incremental risks to the basic interests of participants associated with purely research-related activities do not exceed the incremental risks to the basic interests of individuals associated with those structurally similar social activities" (London 2007a, 594). As interesting as the SEER model is, it is unclear how SEER would make sense of the novel risks associated with *removing stem cells from a healthy eye so as to create a transplant for a damaged eye.* Some research risks may be novel enough that they defy comparison with everyday activities. As such, DSMBs may need to muster their own experience in assessing research risks, as looking to comparator activities may be insufficient.

Wendler and Miller (2008) also attempted to make headway in systematizing research risks. Their target is what they believe is misguided "component analysis," the view that the risks of one intervention in a research study are offset by a clinical benefit of a different intervention in the same study. For example, the risks of a liver biopsy may be justified in a study

because the study also includes an MRI, whose ability to detect an inciden-
tal finding may directly benefit participants by locating a previously undi-
agnosed ailment. The problem with this approach, according to Wendler
and Miller, is that it necessitates that committees such as IRBs adhere to a
"dual track assessment," first asking if an intervention is therapeutic. If the
intervention is not therapeutic, then as long as risks are minimized and
the risks are reasonable compared to the knowledge to be gained, then the
research is ethical. But if the intervention *is* therapeutic, the IRB should
instead ensure that the intervention satisfies equipoise (a discussion of the
concept of *equipoise* and a defense of equipoise as an ethical requirement
in research is included in chapter 4; a discussion of arguments against the
need for equipoise in ethical research is included in chapter 6). Wendler
and Miller do not believe that equipoise is required for ethical research,
so the dual-track assessment that serves as the foundation of component
analysis falls apart.

Additionally, Wendler and Miller hold that the distinction between
"therapeutic" and "non-therapeutic" research is vague and is not supported
by policies such as the Common Rule. They hold that a "direct benefit standard," in which the acceptability of risk is determined by whether participants directly benefit from the research, is also unworkable. On a direct
benefit standard, the CALEC study, designed to examine the feasibility of a
procedure without a primary endpoint of vision being restored to the damaged eye, would not be ethical. Thus, Wendler and Miller move on to a standard they call the "net risks test," which proceeds in a three-step process.

First, the review committees such as the DSMB should examine the risk-
benefit profile of each research intervention and compare those to all available alternatives (which may include no intervention at all). After making
these assessments, the committee can then calculate net risks: "The magnitude of the net risks is a function of the extent to which the intervention
presents increased risks or decreased potential benefits, compared to the
available alternatives" (Wendler and Miller 2008, 509). Per this second step,
the DSMB would determine if the net risks of each intervention are justified by the knowledge gained by the research. Notably, this second step
doesn't require that the research participants themselves directly benefit
from the research. The third step is to then calculate the potential cumulative risks of the study as a whole and determine if those are justified by the
knowledge expected to be gained in the research. If so, then the research is

ethical. Note that according to the net risks test, the *risks above and beyond risks of alternative treatments* are the risks weighed against the gains in generalizable knowledge. In the CALEC study, for example, the net risks for the experimental arm—the CALEC arm—would be expected to be similar, or even less, than those of the CLAU arm. In both cases, the net risk to the damaged eye would be the same in terms of further harm from the surgery or an infection. The net risks from CALEC to the healthy eye may be less than CLAU, given that fewer limbal cells would be taken from the healthy eye in CALEC. Of course, one alternative to CALEC and CLAU is to not opt for surgery at all. Compared to the alternative of doing nothing, the net risks *to the healthy eye* would be greater in CALEC. Are those net risks to the participant worth the gains in generalizable knowledge? That would be the question posed to the DSMB on this standard.

Once the DSMB was clear on the potential risks of the CALEC study, we reasoned that those potential risks were outweighed by the possible benefits. My recollection is that neither Rid, Emanuel, and Wendler's, nor Wendler and Miller's system for assessing the risks of a study were explicitly employed by the DSMB. The diversity of viewpoints on the board allowed us to undertake a holistic assessment based on the expertise of clinicians, stem cell researchers, statisticians, and an ethicist. The next step was a review of the informed consent document—the definitive statement of the risks, benefits, and procedures that each participant would review before entering the study.

DSMBs and Informed Consent

Informed consent is one of the cornerstones of responsible research practice (Brock 2008). Participants offer their informed consent when they offer affirmative agreement to participate in a study after they have been given all relevant information, their decision is voluntarily based upon their understanding of that information, and they are competent to consent (Brock 2008). Gelinas, Wertheimer, and Miller (2016, 36) recognize that "in general, obtaining consent helps to promote transparency and trust in the research enterprise." "Consent is recognized as morally transformative authorization, making certain activities permissible that would otherwise be wrong" (Grady 2015, 860; see also Wenner 2018).

As stated in chapter 2, my experience on DSMBs for NIH-sponsored studies involved DSMBs reviewing consent forms that were initially vetted by

IRBs and making recommendations for approval before the final review and approval of those consent forms by IRBs. One challenge I've encountered is when the DSMB disagrees with the IRB about the language on an informed consent document. I recall a handful of cases in which I advocated for a streamlined discussion of risks in a consent form so as to promote greater readability, but the IRB wanted a more detailed account of risks. Eckstein engages the question of coordination between IRBs and DSMBs extensively, advocating a "more connected data monitoring framework, including through pre-trial and post-trial information sharing among sponsors, IRBs, and DSMBs, as well as avenues for DSMBs to converse with reviewing IRBs during the course of a trial" (Eckstein 2015, 91–92). Eckstein advocates greater communication between IRBs and DSMBs, including greater transparency about DSMB decision-making and sharing of DSMB reports on interim data analyses. Ideally, this would contribute to greater ethical protections for research participants. Some of Eckstein's assumptions about the expertise of both IRB members and DSMB members may be questioned, however. Eckstein may be overestimating the ethical expertise of IRBs while at the same time underestimating the ethical expertise of DSMB—especially those that have a dedicated ethicist. In cases in which the IRB and DSMB disagree—as Eckstein says, "hopefully this will be a rarity"—it is worth remembering the DSMB is merely recommendatory, such that the IRB can choose not to follow its advice (Eckstein 2015, 98). However, given that the DSMB's membership includes individuals who are chosen because of their expertise about the trial, it would be ideal if the IRB did take the DSMB's recommendations under advisement. Eckstein is correct that when there is a great deal at stake, it may be prudent for the DSMB to not merely include their own recommendations to the IRB, but also to articulate the reasoning behind their recommendations.

At the most basic level, any informed consent document should communicate relevant aspects of a study in language that is clear, transparent, and comprehensible to potential participants. The informed consent document for the CALEC study was fairly straightforward even though the distinction between CLAU and CALEC, as well as the risks, were complex and challenging to communicate.

A perennial ethical issue in research is how to craft consent documents that reflect the true benefits and risks of experimental treatments despite the fact that *learning this information is the objective of the study*. Informed consent documents for research are imperfect for this reason—the potential benefits and risks of the study articles are precisely what is being researched. The risks of CLAU appeared a priori to be greater than those of CALEC because CLAU required a greater quantity of limbal cells taken from the donor eye than CALEC, but the study was undertaken to assess if CALEC was a feasible alternative to CLAU. A definitive assessment of the risks and feasibility of CALEC were unknown and were, in fact, the objects of the study. Although informed consent documents for research participation contain the best estimates of the potential benefits and risks of the research, these are ultimately *best estimates*. Informed consent documents don't always make this clear to participants, instead affecting a greater level of precision about the risks and benefits of a research article than is warranted. The question of how to articulate the risks and benefits of study participation in informed consent documents is well-trod territory and not unique to the role of the DSMB. The ethical dimensions of crafting well-written consent forms and creating videos and other media that are used to inform participants, as well as their content, have been the subject of extensive discussion (Brock 2008; Grady 2017; Cummings and Rowbotham 2017; McConnell and Ashley 2017; Kang 2017; Gelinas, Wertheimer, and Miller, 2016).

An informed consent document isn't the entire story of communicating what is involved in a study. Although obtaining consent from participants in research is typically necessary (see chapter 6 for some notable exceptions and the implications of those exceptions), DSMBs should be careful not to make "the common mistake of confusing the consent form with the process of obtaining informed consent" (Brock 2008, 608). A signed consent form may not be necessary for ethically valid consent in cases in which consent can be obtained via other means. It may not be sufficient either, Brock observes, as new information may emerge that would affect a participant's decision to participate, or a participant's values may evolve, rendering previous consent invalid (Brock 2008). For these reasons, the DSMB may evaluate not only the wording of a consent form but also the process by which that information is conveyed. Who makes initial contact with and reviews the option to enroll with the potential participants—someone who can spend adequate time answering questions, someone who can relate to them and the significant decision they are facing? Where do they discuss the possibility of entering the study—somewhere private where they can ask questions in a free and voluntary way, receive honest answers, and mull a decision? Do participants have an opportunity to discuss their enrollment with friends, family, or other health-care providers? Informed consent shouldn't be "one and done," but it is meant to be an ongoing process. Shared decision-making and taking the time to help participants understand their involvement in studies can promote both understanding of research (Grady 2015) and retention of participants. The DSMB's role is not merely to pore over the consent document as they would any other element of the study, but also to ensure that the process of consent is ethical.

Changes in Risk, Change in Consent

One of the reasons cited for informed consent as an ongoing process is that people change. Memories of what someone had consented to in the past may fade, necessitating a reminder of what was consented to in the past. Participants' preferences, goals, and expectations for research may change over time. Thus, participants should have the opportunity to revisit their role in any research study, ensuring participation is consistent with their authentic choices. Perhaps a participant wasn't an autonomous individual when the research started—by virtue of being medically compromised or a minor— and gained autonomy during the course of the study such that revisiting participation may be appropriate (Berkman, Howard, and Wendler 2018). However, participants may have initially consented when they *were* autonomous but lost some level of autonomy along the way, perhaps owing to dementia or other medical circumstances, which rightly requires both the researcher and the legally authorized representative of the participant to assess the advisability of continued participation.

But what happens when it isn't the *participant* who changes, but the *study* that changes? As potential risks, benefits, or alternatives to test articles emerge, participants may rethink their voluntary participation in a study. Having consented to specific details of a study, the evolution of facts on the ground may occasion the "need for ongoing communication process that allow the incorporation of changing information and changed expectations over time" (Grady 2015, 859). The DSMB has information as data accumulates and has the power to recommend to the sponsors and researchers that they act on that knowledge. Throughout a study, the DSMB examines safety; in addition to ongoing monitoring, the data monitoring plan may call for a formal interim analysis, in which both the efficacy and safety of the treatment arms are assessed. In a summary of a review of cases in which a change of consent form was recommended by DSMBs, DeMets, Furberg, and Friedman found "the examples where interim data about adverse events were shared with participants, it was because the adverse events were either more common or more serious than had been expected, or not previously known and therefore not disclosed by the study protocol and consent form" (2006, 21). The FDA's nonbinding guidance for DMCs says that monitoring boards may recommend "informing current and future study participants of newly identified risks via changes in the consent form and, in some cases, obtaining reconsent of current participants to continued study participation" (U.S. Department of Health and Human Services 2006, 19).

The determination as to whether these "newly identified risks" *exist at all* is often part of a DSMB's deliberations. Whether or not an AE is genuinely caused by a study intervention isn't always obvious. Data can be difficult to parse. Multiple investigators may draw different conclusions as to whether a given AE is expected or unexpected, or whether it is the result of a study article or not the result of a study article. Thus, the data received by the DSMB may be ambiguous as to whether participants in one arm are genuinely at greater possible risk of harm. Additionally, each member of the DSMB may be focused on distinct considerations when evaluating the data.[3] Clinicians may be focused on the biological plausibility of an AE being caused by the trial intervention. Statisticians may be focused on whether a seeming change in risks or benefits is mere statistical noise or a true signal. As an ethicist, my focus is on protecting the interests of study participants, ensuring that their voluntary informed consent to continued participation hasn't been compromised as new information comes to light. The above characterization risks depicting the DSMB as the proverbial group of blind men describing an elephant—with clinicians, statisticians, and ethicists all experiencing something different. This metaphor is misleading, as it puts undue emphasis on each DSMB's members' various interpretations rather than placing the focus on the DSMB members' *common goal*. A more apt metaphor returns to the image in the introduction—the pilot, the copilot, and the flight crew all occupying different roles but working collaboratively to keep the passengers safe on their journey. Each member of the DSMB may emphasize different areas of expertise when interpreting study data, but their goal in interpreting those data as accurately as possible remains the common objective of keeping participants safe.

DSMBs are also charged with reviewing new findings from *other studies they are not monitoring*, findings they are altered to by study sponsors, in case new information affects the feasibility or advisability of continuing the study. Per the FDA, "release of results of a related study may have implications for the design of the ongoing study, or even its continuation" (US Health and Human Services 2006, 20). Echoing the FDA, DeMets, Furberg, and Friedman (2006) call this "external information," demonstrating that the publication of external information that shows a clear benefit or harm of an experimental intervention in *another* study should compel a DSMB to rethink the study they are monitoring. The European Medicines Agency both notes the importance of such information and cautions against DMCs acting too hastily in light of such information (EMA 2005, 5): "As the release of study results from other clinical trials in the same area as an ongoing trial monitored by a DMC might impact this trial, such information might be taken into consideration by the DMC. However, such external information should be assessed very carefully and a decision to stop or modify a clinical trial on external information should be taken under exceptional circumstances only."

DSMB meetings may include a review of new journal articles the sponsor has identified that may affect the study. As a purely hypothetical example, if another study team discovered and published results that showed that CLAU was a far better option than CALEC during the CALEC study, this information would have affected the advisability of continuing the trial. If a test article under study is simultaneously being tested in other clinical trials, this creates the possibility that additional risks may be evidenced not just from the study the DSMB is reviewing, but from a host of other studies.

This is one reason London and Kimmelman advocate for the review not of isolated studies, but of "study portfolios," which are a "series of trials that are interrelated by a common set of objectives" (London and Kimmelman 2019, 32). Although the "study portfolio" has its strengths, it is possible this type of sharing of information across multiple studies by a monitoring committee could compromise the objectivity of the analysis; this practice is not without drawbacks (U.S. Department of Health and Human Services 2006, 21). The DSMB may decide to recommend that a study continue yet may conclude that the new information could change the circumstances under which participants might enroll, or stay, in a study. It may be the case that a DSMB, charged with oversight of multiple projects, learns about the risks of a new therapy in one trial, which has application for another trial over which that DSMB also has oversight (Gordon, Sugarman, and Kass 1998). As data are amassed about the efficacy of different treatments, or AEs, the DSMB may recommend a revision of consent forms for newly enrolling participants or create a consent addendum for currently enrolled participants. According to Joffe and Truog (2008, 255), "Respect for subjects would ordinarily include access to interim findings"—an ethical requirement upheld by passing along new data that may affect a participant's willingness to remain in the study. Since the DSMB is the first body to examine new data that might necessitate a revision to consent forms, it is uniquely charged with communicating to sponsors, researchers, or the IRB of record the recommendation that a revision to consent may be necessary.

In some cases in which a consent revision is recommended by the DSMB, participants are given new consent forms. In others, the participants may be given an addendum to a consent form, updating volunteers on targeted and specific aspects of the study. Which of these options is preferable may be a function of the quantity of new information that needs to be conveyed. Here again, there may be disagreements among members of the DSMB, with clinicians, statisticians, and ethicists falling on different sides with respect not only to whether new information should be conveyed but also to which information should be conveyed. Regardless of whether a new consent form, or an addendum, is recommended by the DSMB, the practical complexities of updating consent in multisite trials are enormous. Prior to the 2018 Common Rule revision that allowed the move to a single IRB for multisite trials, if a DSMB recommended a change to a consent form that change would also require approval by each local IRB before participants were informed of new, potentially important information about their participation (Klitzman 2015, 135). The Common Rule revision means it is now less cumbersome to request consent updates. But it is still the case that if a DSMB recommends a change to consent, at least one IRB needs to sign off before the revision is conveyed to participants. Enrollment or administration of experimental treatment may be temporarily halted until revised information is communicated. The temporary suspension is called for because it would be unethical to enroll participants or continue to expose them to risky procedures without their consent incorporating all that is known about the experimental treatment. This temporary suspension may itself be harmful to research participants. The greater the number of research sites, the greater amount of time is needed to communicate new information. Thus, the DSMB is in a position of weighing *the importance of communicating important information* against the *possibility of slowing the study and/or increasing potential risks to participants by virtue of the DSMB's recommendation.*

Slowing a study isn't merely a question of inconveniencing researchers or increasing costs when a study takes longer than planned. If a study ends up taking too long, then generalizable data meant to be produced from the study takes longer and longer to amass. Conceivably, delays could render a study entirely impracticable, in which case the study is stopped altogether. The SIGHT study, discussed in chapter 5, wasn't stopped because of a delay caused by needing to inform participants of new information; however, SIGHT does illustrate the difficulties that emerge when a study is stopped. Stopping a trial, even when that stoppage is warranted, means each enrolled participant was exposed to the risks of entering a trial without the primary benefit—a gain in generalizable knowledge—ever being realized. Thus, delaying a study can have significant ethical implications, utterly disrupting the balance of potential benefits over possible risks.

Even in less extreme cases, in which a study is suspended temporarily, that delay may compromise data collection. Suspicions about the study may be raised among local investigators or participants when they are told to temporarily halt treatment or accrual. Wittes et al. (2007), for example, discuss the concerns of Women's Health Initiative's DSMB that any recommendation—to continue the study, to suspend the study, even to modify consent during the course of the study—would be interpreted by the medical community as telegraphing findings about the risks and benefits of hormone replacement therapy. Wittes et al. recount a drawn-out process that began in fall 1999 of the DSMB recommending informing participants that women enrolled in two of the four trials had higher rates of cardiovascular risk in the treatment arm than the placebo arm. In November of 2002, the DSMB again recommended that the sponsor inform some participants of both a higher instance of stroke and a lower instance of breast cancer in one arm. However, the two members of the DSMB "assigned the task of drafting such a letter were unable to formulate language that would adequately inform the women of the risks and benefits we were observing in a way that would encourage women to continue to participate in the trial" (Wittes et al. 2007, 228). They summarize their discussion by observing, "The decision to recommend informing the participants was a turning point for us. The majority felt that failure to inform the participants would have meant not upholding our pledge to guard their safety and to apprise them in a timely manner of new data that might impact upon their decision to continue in the trial. On the other hand, we all worried lest releasing data from the trial would jeopardize its integrity thereby compromising its ability to influence practice" (Wittes et al. 2007, 231). The questions that arise when DSMBs grapple with recommending reconsent of participants are real world and taxing and can impact the continuation of a trial.

Although the DSMB has a duty to recommend revisions to consent documents when called for, interest in maintaining the integrity of the study for the sake of current participants, and future patients, weighs against time-consuming and cumbersome updating of consent documents. Participants do have autonomy rights to be told information that may affect their continued participation. At the same time, changes to informed consent content may harm the study in the long run. The DSMB's responsibilities here are significant: Even in cases in which voluntary participants have an autonomy right to relevant information, it may not be an easy call to recommend that information be conveyed.

Revising Consent in the Middle of a Study: A Complex Moral Calculation

For bioethicists, especially those with professional backgrounds in philosophy, the below discussion, with its back-and-forth dialectic, may be familiar territory. For those initially learning about the role of ethicists on DSMBs, and how it is that an ethicist approaches complex moral questions, this discussion offers a demonstration of the way in which ethicists have been trained to approach moral questions. In many cases, the role of an ethicist is not to advocate for a particular answer but instead to illustrate the complexity of the question at hand.

Imagine this scenario: Participants with a bacterial infection are enrolled in a study to test a new antibiotic.[4] After receiving the antibiotic, participants are followed for twenty-four weeks, both to see if infection clears up in the first few weeks and to see if they experience any AEs over the next six months. The study drug is expected to have the risk of an itchy, uncomfortable rash in fewer than 1 percent of participants. This possible AE is reported in the consent form all participants sign. This rash isn't expected to be an SAE, but given that it is itchy and uncomfortable, it is expected to be at least a "moderate" AE. The 1 percent figure isn't arbitrarily chosen—it may be based on animal studies, phase I studies, or on the frequency of rashes from similar antibiotics. Thus, although there isn't absolute certainty about the potential risk of the rash, the consent document reviewed by the DSMB reflects the best information known prior to the commencement of the study. The DSMB plans an interim analysis of the data at six months, unless a large number of SAEs require an earlier meeting.

Per the Common Rule, all unanticipated AEs or protocol deviations are reported to the IRB: there needs to be "prompt reporting to the IRB" of any "unanticipated problems involving risks to subjects or others or any serious or continuing noncompliance" with the Common Rule or IRB determinations (§46.108.4(i)). Since the rash is an expected AE when using this antibiotic—and not an "unexpected problem"—it is possible that investigators don't communicate information about the rash to the IRB at all. The IRB receives word of AEs if and when they trickle in, whereas the DSMB sees the aggregate data about AEs, expected or not, and not just individual incidents as they take place. The DSMB learns at the interim analysis meeting that the cumulative rate of getting the rash in the experimental arm is closer to 10 percent, not the expected 1 percent per the consent form. After much discussion among the members of the DSMB, the clinicians are convinced of the biological plausibility of the rash being caused by the study article, the statisticians are convinced that there is a clear statistical signal, and the ethicist has questions as to whether the continued voluntary participation of the people in the study is compromised by not being told this new information. The DSMB must now make a determination as to what to do next.

The first question the DSMB might consider is whether to recommend suspending the study, perhaps pending more information about the rash or its frequency. The rash is an expected, but not serious, AE, and although it is itchy and uncomfortable, it is less harmful than the bacterial infections the antibiotic is designed to treat, so there is no need to recommend stopping the study. Even though the likelihood of getting the rash is tenfold higher than the researchers and the DSMB initially thought, the DSMB advocates continuing the study because the potential balance of benefits over risks remains favorable. The potential benefits of the antibiotic still outweigh the risks of this moderate AE.

A second question the DSMB considers is whether new information about the rash should be communicated to participants. If the sole consideration is the autonomy rights of voluntary participants to be informed, then this is an easy call: The DSMB should recommend a revision of the consent form for as-yet unenrolled participants and a consent addendum for currently enrolled participants so as to best inform both newly enrolled participants and current participants of the elevated risk of harm from the trial drug. The study commenced before all the information was available about the study drug and the risk of this moderate AE. Now that new information is available, it stands to reason this should be communicated to participants. Another way to look at the question is this: If the study were starting now, at the point that the DSMB has knowledge that the risk of rash is 10 percent, is there any possible justification for *not communicating* that risk to potential participants? Of course not.

Now imagine a situation in which the data do not straightforwardly indicate that a revised consent form and addendum are indicated. The data received by the DSMB do not merely show that the risk of the rash is 10 percent. Instead, it appears that the likelihood of the rash from the study drug is attenuated by time. Within the first week of receiving the study drug, the risk of getting the rash is fairly high. But as time goes on, the risk dissipates, such that by the twenty-four-week closeout visit, no participant who hasn't already experienced the rash presents with a rash reasonably expected to be caused by the new antibiotic.[5]

The DSMB has a more complex role than to merely recommend that new information be communicated to the participants. To understand the complexity of the situation, it should be made clear that after the DSMB initially reviewed the protocol, it is highly unlikely that all participants enrolled simultaneously. If the study was conducted at multiple sites, each of those sites may have taken more, or less, time to initiate recruitment. Even if the study was taking place at a single site, it is still highly unlikely that the number of participants needed to adequately power the study so as to find a statistically significant signal about the efficacy of this new antibiotic *all came to that single site on a single day*. The likely scenario is that even though the study follows participants for six months, it might take at least

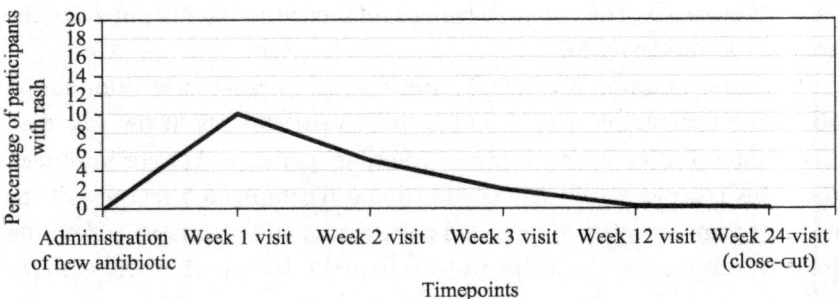

Figure 3.1
Incidence of rash over time in treatment arm

that long, or even longer, to enroll all the participants in the study. Some participants would agree to be in the study shortly after it began enroll-ment. Others may enroll weeks, or months, later. Some participants would be nearing their final closeout visit on the same day other participants are just signing their consent to begin the study.

Understanding the complexity of informing participants about this newly discovered AE considers that different participants will be at different stages of the study at the same time. *New enrollees* should be given informa-tion about the 10 percent risk of the AE. But what about those participants who are at the twelve- or twenty-week mark—still in the study, but well past the "danger zone" of being likely to get a rash from the antibiotic?

Here, "consent as an ongoing process" is more complex than merely conveying the same information to all participants. What it means to offer consent to different participants may vary based on the stage at which the participant is in the study. The participant who has yet to be randomized should be told about the 10 percent chance of the rash. The participant who is at the twenty-week mark, who took the antibiotic five months ago, is unlikely to get a rash at this point. Telling the participant who is at the twenty-week mark they have a 10 percent chance of getting a rash is mis-leading and might unnecessarily worry them. The data show the risk of getting a rash at the twenty-week mark isn't 10 percent. Communicating to the participant who has been in the study for twenty weeks "the risk of rash from the antibiotic is 10%" is likely to be misconstrued. What is gained by telling a research participant new information that doesn't pertain to their situation and will only cause anxiety?

Researchers may worry participants will withdraw from the study and thus may balk at DSMB recommendations motivated by protecting the safety of participants (Resnik 2009). Herson (2017, 141) remarks on the possibility of trial withdrawals in light of informed consent revisions: "It is possible that some patients will refuse to sign the modified informed consent and drop out of the trial. This is their right. That this, or reduced compliance . . . might be a consequence of reconsenting should not be part of the discussion of whether or not to reconsent." The DSMB may recommend to the IRB that newly randomized participants, and those within one week of getting the new treatment, should be told about the potential 10 percent risk. Participants who are outside that window should be told that there is new information that has potentially altered the likelihood of a risk of harm and, for this reason, they are urged to attend their twelve- and twenty-four-week visits. But to tell those participants that they have a 10 percent chance of a rash is inaccurate and potentially harmful. Telling patients that they have this high a likelihood of getting a rash, when they really don't, would *contribute* to the possible risks of the study by exacerbating stress or anxiety. Recall the risk of stress or anxiety during the CALEC trial, when participants were in a "wait and see mode" as their limbal stem cell grafts grew (or not) in the lab. Telling participants that something may or may not happen, but they just have to wait until the researcher knows more, can be anxiety provoking even if no physical harm happens in the meantime. The analogy here is imperfect—more hung in the balance for the CALEC patients, who faced a monumental next step rather than a rash that was judged to be a "moderate" AE. However, in both cases, the lesson is the same: heightened stress or anxiety should be taken seriously as a harm.

A response on the part of those who would advocate a reconsenting process in the study of the antibiotic may be that participants have a right to all information about the experimental treatment. Why inform some participants but not others? Arguments from autonomy for informed consent support the claim that *all* participants should be told *all* information pursuant to a study. Furthermore, given that there is no compelling reason to say that the participants at the twenty-week mark have less autonomy than at the one-week mark (all have already received the experimental antibiotic—they are all equally unable to go back in time to revisit their participation), then what the week-one participant and the week-twenty participant are told should be the same.

Bolstering this position is the claim that it would be ethically questionable that different information is conveyed to different participants who are all enrolled in the same study. All participants should have their autonomy equally respected, which means that everyone should be given the same information when they enroll in the study. According to Herson (2017, 141), "It is not considered good practice to show (a) modified consent form only to new patients entering the trial." There may be reasons to alter the *consent process*—perhaps giving the information to different subjects in their respective native languages or adjusting information for reading level, including appropriate assent language for young children rather than autonomous adults, and so on. But even if the way information is conveyed is different for different participants, *the information itself* shouldn't be different. Selectively conveying information to some participants, but not others, is a violation of autonomy.

This argument from autonomy, while compelling when the study is initiated, weakens as the study progresses. The DSMB may be guided not only by protecting the autonomy of participants but also by the need to maximize the most favorable balance of potential benefits over risks. The as-yet enrolled subjects have a right to make a decision based on all available information. However, as time progresses, there is little to be gained communicating information to participants that doesn't apply to them. It is possible that conveying information that may upset participants, yet doesn't apply to them, will harm them. Thus, the DSMB rightly should advocate communicating different information to different subjects.

What of the objection to this position that the DSMB is exercising benign paternalism by withholding new information it receives from participants? After all, no one can go back in time and "untake" the antibiotic. Why pass along *any* new information to any participant, at any stage in the study? If the treatment window has already passed, and nothing can be done about the possibility of the rash, why bother telling any participant? Is the focus on maximizing a potential balance of benefits over risks embraced by the DSMB an ethic that proves too much, in that it supports failure to pass along *any* new information?

This concern fails to take into consideration that the one-week or twenty-week participant is still in follow-up. Communicating the information to participants about potential AEs may cause anxiety. However, it may also compel some participants to attend their final closeout appointment, which is a positive consequence of newly communicated information. A direct benefit to participants may result from communicating this information; thus the DSMB is right to advocate for a consent addendum even for the participants who are nearing the end of the follow-up window. Notice, however, that the response to this objection doesn't necessitate that those participants who are beyond the closeout appointment need to be further informed. The ethic that guides DSMB decision-making doesn't require that the post-study participant needs to be told because there is nothing that can be gained, medically or psychologically, from communicating this potential AE. Note, however, that the necessity to follow-up after the end of this study doesn't indicate that post-study follow-up might not be indicated in other studies. Given the severity of some AEs, post-study follow-up may be indicated in some trials with interventions that pose significant risks. According to DeMets, Furberg, and Friedman (2006, 34), "Although post-trial follow-up is uncommon, if [sic] may be important in selected situations. Usually, it will be the investigators who make the decision for follow up. But the monitoring committee may help to identify particular instances."

There is an important lesson learned from the claim that it isn't incumbent upon the research team to communicate about the rash to participants after this study is completed. This underscores the focus of a positive balance of potential benefits over potential risks that guides DSMBs and clinical research. If autonomy were the paramount ethical principle in research ethics, then it wouldn't matter if the participant received the antibiotic one week ago, twenty weeks ago, or thirty weeks ago—the person has a "right to be informed." But whether they should be informed is not about current or former participants' rights—it is about what can be gained from communicating the information. This observation is one that will be elaborated upon in chapter 6, which examines the ethical framework that guides DSMB decision-making.

The ethicist on the DSMB has a role in helping to compose or review any new informed consent document or addendum, but the ethicist's expertise may also be helpful in drawing out the above distinctions for clinicians and statisticians on the committee, analyzing the back-and-forth of the ethical arguments on each side of controversial issues, such as when to disclose additional information as part of the consent process. The clinicians and statisticians have an important role interpreting the data about the risks of

the antibiotic, communicating those data in ways that are clear to everyone on the DSMB, explaining the clinical impact of this AE on participants,
the biological plausibility that a given AE is caused by the study article and
the likelihood that a true statistical signal exists. They also have an essential
role in interpreting the data in trials more complex than the simple two-arm,
twenty-four-week trial, expected to have at most moderate AEs, discussed
above. Distinct trial types (one-armed trials, two-arm unblinded trials, two-
arm blinded trials, pragmatic trials (Weijer and Taljaard 2024), among many
other types of trials) as well as the complexity of data analysis (early false
signals, chance imbalances in randomization, weighing possible benefits
against risks) only increase the complications surrounding consent adden-
dums or reconsent of participants. Clinicians and statisticians offer their
candid assessment of how the study's unique properties affect the participants in the trial. The ethicist on the DSMB uses those insights to uphold
ethical standards when, for example, some participants but not others need
to be given additional information over the course of a study. The ethicist
helps to ensure that the subtleties of conveying the data amassed by scientists can be conveyed to participants in a clear and helpful manner without
leading to further harm.

Conclusion

Weighing of potential risks against benefits in clinical research and communicating those via informed consent is well-trod territory in research ethics. But DSMBs take on a special role, one that adds greater depth to these
discussions. When it comes to assessing potential risks and benefits, the
DSMB comprises experts in the area under study who are uniquely qualified to evaluate possible risks and benefits. Even still, as illustrated in the
CALEC trial, recognizing and weighing risks can be a challenge for DSMB
members. The CALEC trial illustrates how the assessment of research risk
can be counterintuitive, even to clinicians who are familiar with the study
procedures. A robust back-and-forth among DSMB members before a study
begins can help to clarify a study's risks.

Once potential risks are appropriately understood, the DSMB reviews the
consent form and consent process, making recommendations to the IRB
that ultimately approves them, in order to ensure that potential risks will
be communicated effectively to participants. The contours of informed

consent—its strengths, weaknesses, and methods for improving informed consent—are similarly well-trod territory. The unique role of the DSMB emerges when questions arise *during* the course of a study about changing risk profiles. Since the DSMB is positioned to learn of additional risks across multiple sites, and how they are weighed against the perceived benefits of the study, the DSMB makes an informed recommendation whether participants should offer additional consent to participation. The decision to "re-consent" participants isn't a straightforward one, however. DSMBs must weigh the autonomy rights of participants to be informed and to make voluntary decisions based upon that information against the possible risks associated with that "re-consent." This is not a one-size-fits-all decision, as the logistics of undertaking a new consent procedure, the nature of the new risks, the unique circumstances of individual participants, and the possible impact on the study as a whole, must be taken into account. DSMB members weigh these considerations, recognizing that respecting the autonomy of participants may mean different processes for different individuals. Just as initial consent may take different forms depending on the age, cognitive capacity, literacy, or other considerations about participants, so too the "re-consent" process may take different forms for different participants based on their unique circumstances. The singular role of the DSMB necessitates a singular set of responsibilities when upholding informed consent for research.

There are cases, though, when merely communicating to participants new information about potential risks isn't enough. Recall that the novel antibiotic case began, "The first question the DSMB might consider is whether to recommend suspending the study." The focus of this chapter was evaluating potential risks and the pros and cons of "re-consenting" participants; the option of recommending suspension of the study wasn't explored. Some trials may require greater involvement by the DSMB—recommendations of suspension or, in the most extreme cases, closure. The circumstances that lead to these extreme measures are the subject of the next chapter.

The macula is the center portion of the retina, responsible for fine vision (such as reading the words on this page). If the macula is displaced by fluid in the eye called the "vitreous" the macula can become distorted, compromising vision. This displacement, or pulling, is called "macular traction." If macular traction results in a hole in the macula then this macular hole can also compromise vision. It may be possible to exert a small amount of pressure on the vitreous, pushing the macula back into its proper shape, correcting the distortion or closing the macular hole. This pressure could come from injecting a small amount of gas (air) into the vitreous. The injection of the gas is called "pneumonic vitreolysis," and the gas used in this type of procedure is perfluoropropane. Protocol AG was a randomized clinical trial designed to test if pneumonic vitereolysis could correct macular traction. Protocol AH was a single-arm study to determine if pneumonic vitereolysis could close a macular hole. "An independent data and safety monitoring committee (DSMC) provided oversight and recommended halting enrollment into both studies on February 11, 2020, after review of the combined data from Protocols AG and AH on the incidence of rhegmatogenous retinal detachments and retinal tears" (Chan et al. 2021, 1593).

Equipoise as a Mainstay of DSMB Work

Many participants in clinical research are in randomized trials—trials in which participants are randomly assigned their future experience in the study. In those randomized trials, participants consent to being in the study, but they don't consent to a specific intervention. Rather, they consent to a set of possible interventions and then are randomly assigned to one of those. Those random assignments, or arms of the study, might include an experimental intervention, the standard of care, or placebo. It is important for those assignments to be randomized to reduce bias in the study (Joffe and Truog 2008): Given a choice of arms, participants may choose one arm over the other based on characteristics that could affect the success of treatment, such as participants' education level, ability to adhere to the study arm, or social support. Thus, randomization is one step toward ensuring the results of the study are not compromised by methodological bias. The assumption is that although participants haven't consented to *a particular arm* of the study, their autonomy is still respected if they offer consent to being randomized into *any one of the arms*, so long as they understand the procedures in each arm and the concept of randomization. Since participants don't choose the arm of the study to which they are assigned, it is crucial to monitor the study to ensure that no one is disadvantaged, or misses out on an advantage, by virtue of the arm to which they were assigned. As studies progress, DSMBs may recommend changes to ensure this balance of advantage and disadvantage are maintained. The FDA's nonbinding recommendations for data and safety monitoring committees state that during the course of a trial, committees may recommend changing eligibility criteria, altering dosage levels, or employing methods to screen out participants who during the course of a trial have been found to be at a greater risk of harm (U.S. Department of Health and Human Services 2006, 19). DSMBs should be cautious in advocating for extensive changes, for fear of either biasing the researchers by telegraphing how the trial is progressing, as discussed in the previous chapter, or by violating the integrity of the trial. It is the purview of DSMBs to oversee studies and recommend changes to promote participant safety, but DSMBs need to proceed with caution to ensure that no one is disadvantaged, or misses out on an advantage, by virtue of being in a trial. Studies in which no one is disadvantaged, or misses out on an advantage, are said to be in *equipoise*.

A foundational ethical assumption guiding DSMB work is that clinical trials should commence and continue only if they are in equipoise. DeMets, Furberg, and Freidman summarize the obligations of the DSMB with respect to equipoise as follows:

> The trial must begin in a position of clinical equipoise. That is, the informed scientific and medical communities do not know which of the approaches being tested in the trial is preferable. As the data begin to accumulate, the monitoring committee may decide that the trends in the primary outcome are so strong in one direction or another (i.e., in favor or against the new intervention) that clinical equipoise is no longer tenable and the study must be stopped before its scheduled end. The study has achieved its goal of providing an answer. (2005, 8)

Similarly, London observes among frameworks that guide clinical research, "One of the most promising frameworks holds that as a necessary condition for ethically acceptable human-subjects research, clinical trials must begin in and be designed to disturb a state of equipoise" (London 2007a, 572). Freedman holds that "equipoise is an ethically necessary condition in all cases of clinical research" (Freedman 1987, 141). If a clinical trial commences that isn't in equipoise, the trial was not ethical to begin with because some participants were disadvantaged or unduly advantaged by virtue of the arm into which they were initially randomized. "It is unethical to randomize if available data show convincingly that one arm of the proposed study would yield significantly greater benefit than the other. Moreover, while a randomized trial may have been ethical when designed, interim finding may influence whether it is ethical for the trial to continue" (Gordon, Sugarman, and Kass 1998, 1).

The import and controversy surrounding a study's equipoise can be illustrated by opposing views of the SUPPORT trial, which compared the effectiveness of two levels of oxygen given to premature babies. Lantos and Feudtner say that the "first concern" about the trial rested "on a belief that, when the SUPPORT study was being designed, the state of medical knowledge was already sufficiently clear about the optimal amount of oxygen to give premature babies and that therefore any study of differing oxygen therapy protocols was unnecessary and unethically exposed infants to a treatment known to be inferior" (Lantos and Feudtner 2015, 30). If SUPPORT had been designed such that some oxygen levels were known to be inferior, the study would not have been in equipoise and thus would have been unethical.[1] However, it is argued that SUPPORT wasn't unethical because "when the study began, targeting an oxygen-saturation range of 85 to 95% was becoming standard clinical practice, and the American Academy of Pediatrics (AAP) later recommended this range in its 2007 guidelines. The SUPPORT researchers and institutional review boards (IRBs), practicing clinicians, and the AAP had no scientific evidence to expect a difference in mortality between the two treatment groups in SUPPORT—one with the oxygen saturation target of 85 to 89%, the other with the target of 91 to 95%" (Hudson, Guttmacher, and Collins 2013, 2350). Hudson, Guttmacher, and Collins recount the scientific foundations for the SUPPORT trial, as well as a passage in the informed consent document that "describes the clinical equipoise at the time of the study, which was, in fact, the justification for conducting a clinical trial" (Hudson, Guttmacher, and Collins 2013, 2351). The point here is not to relitigate the ethics of the SUPPORT trial but rather to illustrate the high stakes and ethical debates surrounding questions of equipoise.[2]

Even if a trial begins in equipoise, if the trial falls out of equipoise while in progress, then it should be stopped because participants become disadvantaged or are deprived of a relative advantage by continuance in the study. If a study is stopped early, the knowledge gained from the study could benefit future patients sooner. If a study is stopped early because it fell out of equipoise, patients are less likely to be exposed to treatments that are ineffective or may have the opportunity to access treatments that are effective. "If large and statistically significant differences in important outcomes are apparent during a trial, it may be appropriate to terminate a trial early, minimizing risks to subjects and saving resources" (Gordon, Sugarman, and Kass 1998, 2). In most cases, the DSMB is the sole body with access to the entirety of trial data during the course of a study; as such, the DSMB has the responsibility to monitor equipoise in the trial.

DSMBs can recommend that sponsors stop trials that fall out of equipoise, and they have the ethical responsibility to do so. DSMBs "are charged with deciding when the accumulated evidence justified closing the trial. Ideally, the decision to close a trial respects protocol-specified stopping guidelines that function to preserve both the scientific validity and the ethical integrity of the trial" (Joffe and Truog 2008, 251). Joffe and Truog catalogue the circumstances under which a trial may be stopped by the DSMB, such as logistical problems, lack of accrual (a topic discussed in chapter 5), the fact that even if data collection continues, there is little hope of evidence that one arm is better than the other (futility), or the fact that one arm of the study is found to be decidedly inferior or superior to other arms (efficacy). Viele, McGlothlin, and Broglio (2016), as well as the Department of Health and Human Services Inspector General's report (2013), present similar reasons for which a DSMB may recommend a trial be stopped. Equipoise is about the last of two these concerns: in the case of *futility*, the arms are in equipoise and no additional evidence will disrupt that fact; in the case of *efficacy*, one arm has been found to be therapeutically worse or better than another prior to collection of all data. Even when the language of "equipoise" is not explicitly invoked, DSMB members, who debate the trade-offs between continuing a study in which there may be convincing evidence that some participants are harmed by continuing and determining whether there is sufficient evidence to change clinical practice if the study is stopped, are making claims about equipoise. The European Medicines Agency (EMA 2005, 3) begins its discussion of DMCs with this claim: "Clinical trials frequently extend over a long period of time. Thus, for ethical reasons it is desirable to ensure that for patients participating in such trials there is no unavoidable increased risk for harm. On the other hand it is also important to ensure that a trial continues for an adequate period of time and is not stopped too early to answer its scientific questions." The term *equipoise* is not invoked, but the takeaway is clear.

Although regarded as a mainstay of DSMB work, the concept of equipoise is not straightforward. Identification of equipoise is said to have originated in the work of Charles Fried, who argued that an RCT's equipoise is not a sufficient moral justification for waiving informed consent (Fried 2016, 5; see also 58–59, 163). Fried argued the *personal care* owed to a participant in a clinical trial means even if a physician viewed a study to be in equipoise, that did not mean the patient's informed consent was unnecessary. Fried held that patients are entitled to make choices about whether to enroll, or to continue enrollment, in a study "even if we are sure that there is only one rational choice for him to make" (Fried 2016, 56).

Bioethicists spend a great deal of time thinking—some may say overthinking—equipoise in clinical trials. The point of this chapter is not to comprehensively re-interrogate the concept of equipoise or re-interrogate the defense of a DSMB's charge to maintain equipoise both at the commencement, and continuation, of a trial. Both of these tasks have been done previously in bioethics literature. This chapter's discussion of equipoise is styled to first illustrate myriad analyses of the term, with an eye to demonstrating what can be learned from these disparate conceptions. The goal is not to settle on a single true analysis of the concept of equipoise, but to gain clarity about the monumental charge that DSMBs face when examining the equipoise of a clinical trial. Illustrating diverse notions of equipoise highlights the complexity of the DSMB's responsibilities. The second discussion—the defense of the ethical imperative DSMBs are faced with in maintaining equipoise—is similarly not designed to be an exhaustive examination of all arguments in favor of maintaining equipoise. Rather, several arguments are classified into one of two types: one that defends equipoise as essential to scientific methodology, and the other that views equipoise as an extension of other imperatives that guide ethical research.

In my years on DSMBs, on diverse committees, and among many impressive clinicians and statisticians with whom I've had the honor to serve, I've never once heard anyone dispute the importance of maintaining equipoise in a clinical trial. There may be debates about whether equipoise was genuinely disrupted, such as in the SUPPORT trial, or if the conclusion that equipoise was disrupted was too hasty. Wittes et al. (2007, 229) observed that stopping the Women's Health Initiative trials "prematurely could mean that the trial would not result in a clinically important answer to the questions it set out to ask." Even within the context of these debates as to whether a study remained in equipoise or not, the ethical significance of equipoise was never in doubt. Statisticians acknowledge, almost with a shrug, that they are taught the concept of equipoise early in their schooling; the centrality of equipoise isn't disputed. It is taken for granted that it is wrong to start a study in which one arm will certainly experience a greater balance of potential risks over benefits, and that once a study commences, if it is found that one arm in fact does experience a greater balance of risks over benefits, it is unethical to continue. Arguments about what precisely equipoise is, or whether it should be maintained, take place among philosophers and philosophically trained bioethicists. In my admittedly anecdotal experience, others who serve on DSMBs rarely engage these questions.

Although maintaining equipoise is viewed by many as a mainstay of DSMB work, complexities about what equipoise is, and arguments on both sides for maintaining equipoise in clinical trials, persist among bioethicists. Examining competing analyses of the concept of equipoise is the first step in understanding the difficulties DSMBs face in their charge to maintain equipoise and why this disputed concept is nonetheless viewed as a cornerstone of DSMB practice.

Competing Analyses of Equipoise

There are numerous accounts of what equipoise means in the bioethics literature.[3] Discussions of competing accounts can be found in London (2007a) and Joffe and Truog (2008). Below are only a few proposals, numbered to make comparisons easier to follow:

E1: "Equipoise is the state of being suspended equally between two options." (Veatch 2007, 179)

E2: "Equipoise—the state of uncertainty or lack of grounded preference concerning which of two treatment options is preferable." (Gifford 2007, 135)

E3: "There is consensus that clinical trials should be launched only when there is sufficient promise for the new intervention but insufficient evidence to justify broad use, a condition called equipoise." (Miller and Brody 2007, 155, quoting Brody, McCullough, and Sharp 2005)

E4: "Relative equipoise is the zone within which there is legitimate disagreement about whether one treatment is superior to another from the point of view of the relevant scientists or clinicians." (Veatch 2007, 179)

E5: "A randomized trial is ethical only in circumstances of "clinical equipoise"—a genuine uncertainty within the medical community as to whether . . . any of the . . . treatment arms are superior to the other(s)." (Miller and Brody 2003, 19)

E6: "[Charles] Fried coined the term 'equipoise'" to describe the ethically necessary condition for conducting an RCT: physician-investigators must be indifferent to the therapeutic value of experimental treatments and control treatments evaluated in the trial." (Miller and Brody 2003, 23, citing Fried 2016)

E7: "According to Freedman, an RCT is ethical so long as the professional community has not yet reached a consensus, which recognizes that 'medicine is a social rather than individual in nature.' When, and only when, clinical equipoise is satisfied will patients enrolled in a clinical trial be assured that they will not be randomized to treatments known to be inferior." (Miller and Brody 2003, 24, quoting Freedman 1987)

Veatch's claim in E1, that equipoise is the state of being equally suspended between two options, is a good launching point for discussion. Although E1 might, at first glance, appear to be a two-place relation, on further examination, E1 is a three-place relation: A is in a state of being equally suspended between options x and y. Veatch's minimalist conception demonstrates how many questions about equipoise are yet to be answered: What are those options, x and y, that are equally poised? Options x and y are poised between A, but who, or what, is A? Notice also that E1 is a metaphysical claim, and not an epistemic one: Whatever equipoise is according to E1, it is a claim about reality, about two options (x and *y*, as yet unnamed) which are *not merely perceived, believed, or known to be* equally suspended, but which *actually are* equally suspended.

E2 marks a departure from this metaphysical claim. Gifford conceives of equipoise in terms of "uncertainty" or "lack of grounded preference." This echoes the Department of Health and Human Services Inspector General's report (2013, 1): "DSMBs approach trial monitoring with uncertainty regarding whether the intervention or drug being tested will be superior to existing treatments or at all effective until proven otherwise." Both of these are epistemic claims—claims not necessarily about what is true in the world, but instead claims about what is believed or known to be true. The disjunction between "uncertainty" and "lack of grounded preference" is interesting, as one can have the former without the later, and vice versa. I can be *uncertain* after losing my keys (yet again) as to where my keys are, but I unquestionably *prefer* that my keys are somewhere in the house. I can have *no grounded preference* which restaurant my family takes me to for my birthday (for the umpteenth time, I don't care where we go as long as I don't have to do the dishes), but I can be *certain* that if my husband chooses, it will be a steakhouse. The three-place relationship here is about a lack of certainty or preference—A is uncertain about preferring x to y, A has no grounded preference between x and y—which means that A must be some agent, some individual capable of certainties or preferences. But who A is remains an open question. Finally, E2 expands on what options x and y are—namely, treatment options.

E3's take on the comparison between x and y is that one of them is a "new intervention," and implicitly, the other is an intervention (or perhaps, lack thereof) that isn't new. Tacitly, this newness consists of being a new treatment for a particular condition under study, but not necessarily a novel treatment that had never before been used or tested. For example, as discussed in chapter 2, rituximab was tested as a new therapy for acute exacerbations of IPF, but that doesn't necessitate that rituximab had been developed specifically for the STRIVE-IPF trial. Rituximab had been in use for other conditions; its use for acute exacerbations of IPF in STRIVE was new. E3 continues with the notion that equipoise is an epistemic assessment: the points of comparison between x and y are about "sufficient promise" vs. "insufficient evidence." In making a claim that the new intervention has "sufficient promise," the implication is that equipoise requires that trial arms aren't proposed willy-nilly. "Sufficient promise" goes beyond mere uncertainty or lack of preference. Before launching a trial using human participants, a new intervention should be likely to work, based on earlier studies, animal studies, or evidence of the intervention having been used elsewhere. One of the duties of DSMBs if they are called upon to convey recommendations to a sponsor before a trial begins is to examine the background and justification for the trial. DSMBs are protocol specific, well versed in the field, and familiar with its literature and clinical practices. With respect to protocols AG and AH, for example, pneumonic vitereolysis had been previously used by some practitioners to correct macular traction or close macular holes; thus, clinical trials AG and AH, which might *demonstrate* its efficacy, were warranted. E3 adds a new component to the discussion, claiming that "clinical trials should be launched only" when equipoise has obtained. This "should" is a moral claim: it is morally unjustified to launch a clinical trial unless initially there is equipoise among the arms of the trial. Miller and Brody do not necessarily endorse this moral claim, as discussed in chapter 6, but they correctly attribute this moral claim to many individuals.

Veatch, in E4, proposes a more complex notion of equipoise. Veatch introduces a claim as to who A might be—the "relevant scientists or clinicians." In general, the term "relevant" is a tricky one, as it is difficult to pin down what counts as relevance. Claims about relevance are often circular: certain properties or attributes single out "relevant" expertise, while at the same time, "relevant" expertise involves having those very properties or attributes. Another potential complicating factor is Veatch's claim that equipoise is not merely a claim that "x is believed to be superior to y," or vice versa, but rather that "x is in a zone of superiority." The reference to a "zone of superiority" may be a practical improvement, insofar as it allows for certain types of trial design, such as noninferiority trials. Noninferiority trials typically proceed with a "margin of inferiority"—a range in which treatment x can be *close enough* in terms of efficacy to treatment y, in order for x to be judged "not inferior" to y. For example, if one medication entirely clears up a rash in ten days, and another medication entirely clears up the same rash in fourteen days, that four-day difference may not be sufficient to say that the second medication is truly inferior to the first. Both do the job equally well; one merely takes a few days longer. Hence, the "non-inferiority margin" can be understood as a range, or a zone. Veatch's

definition proposes we understand equipoise not in terms of absolute superiority or inferiority of x to y, but rather within a range.

Meeting or exceeding a noninferiority margin may be one of the pre-
specified endpoints in the trial; as such, it is scientists and clinicians who
make the assessment as to what the noninferiority margin is in a given study.
Confoundingly, for some patients or research participants, what they may
perceive as "inferior" treatments may nonetheless fall within the "noninferiority margin." A medication that is *not quite* as efficacious may be determined to fall within the "noninferiority margin" of a given study. In such a
case, the medication may be "inferior" in one sense but "noninferior" for the
sake of clinical practice. The stipulation of "noninferiority" may make sense
to researchers but may not be convincing to all patients. Acuna, Chesney,
and Baxter (2019, 305) in their discussion of patient preferences in non nfe-
riority trials, point out, "Expert opinion is used to interpret the importance
of treatment differences, although this approach may not be a valid and
reliable reflection of what matters to patients. Patients and clinicians often
have different preferences for treatments and choose different trade-offs
when deciding between various treatment options." A rash medication that
is equally efficacious in fourteen days may be clinically "noninferior" to
one that works in ten days. However, distinctions about the time the treatment takes to work, the cost of treatment, or the burden on the patient to
take one type of treatment (such as an oral medication) rather than another
(an IV treatment that can only be administered at a clinic) can have a real-
world impact as to which treatment is "inferior" in the eyes of patients. One
can imagine a scenario in which a patient cares deeply about clearing up
that rash four days earlier—in time for the big wedding, the job interview,
the audition. "Clinician-investigators might be indifferent with respect to
the trial's 'hard' endpoints—mortality or major morbidity—but prospective trial participants are likely to consider factors such as quality of life
and practical burdens as well" (Joffe and Truog 2008, 249). Those quality-
of-life and "practical burdens" may be of lasting significance to patients
and participants. For this reason, Acuna, Chesney, and Baxter (2019, 306)
conclude, "Given the critical nature of the ΔNI [noninferiority margin] in
the design and interpretation of noninferiority trials, there is a need to consider patient preferences, particularly because patients and clinicians have
different preferences for treatment and have shown different trade-offs
when deciding between various treatment options." Yet according to E4, the

determination of "the zone of equivalency" falls to the scientists and clinicians studying x and y, not to the research participants or patients who are taking x or y. This focus on scientists and clinicians, rather than patients or research participants, is a troubling exclusion, one DSMB members should flag in their communication to researchers. Joffe and Truog (2008) observe that attributions of equipoise can differ with respect to whether it is physicians and investigators who are making the determination, versus patients and participants, and whether the determination is made by individuals or communities, a point further explored in chapter 5. Hence, there can be 1) individual (physician-investigator) equipoise, 2) individual (patient-participant) equipoise, 3) clinical equipoise among the professional community, or 4) community equipoise among the community of patients and participants. E4 is an example of the third type.

E5 makes a stronger claim than E4. Rather than embracing the notion of a "zone" of superiority, here Miller and Brody assert a claim about actual superiority. Veatch may mean something distinct by "relative equipoise" in E4 than what Miller and Brody are calling "clinical equipoise" in E5; it may be that E4 and E5 are engaging different concepts. Miller and Brody attribute to some theorists this epistemic notion of equipoise—equipoise in E5 is about "genuine uncertainty." Finally, E5 claims that the party A, in this state of genuine uncertainty, is the "medical community." Is the medical community understood as the relevant scientists and clinicians cited above in E4, which would include the DSMB members? Perhaps. One thing is clear in both E4 and E5: The individual, or individuals A, who are making judgments about equipoise are *not* patients or research participants. As stated above, this is a significant lacuna. E1, E2, and E3, in not specifying who is equally suspended, uncertain, or has no preference between x and y, leave the door open that patients or research participants may be in a state of equipoise. E4 and E5 foreclose that possibility.

E6 incorporates several of the above observations: Equipoise is an ethical requirement of clinical trials, x and y are experimental treatments and control treatments (including a placebo, if appropriate), and A includes physician-investigators. Both E5 and E6 don't distinguish between the ethical necessity of a trial *starting* from a state of equipoise and the ethical necessity of a trial *remaining* in equipoise. According to E6, A is not the medical community as a whole, but instead the physician-investigators engaged in the RCT comparing x and y. Hence, E6 captures what Benjamin Freedman

called "theoretical equipoise," an individual investigator A's lack of preference of x over y, not a consensus that there is a lack of treating preference
within the medical community. Freedman distinguished "theoretical equipoise" with indifference among "the expert clinical community," which
he called "clinical equipoise" (Freedman 1987). Whether or not indifference is disrupted among the clinical community is of lasting importance.
If a study is believed to fall out of equipoise by the researchers, but the
data aren't convincing to the medical community as a whole, then the
study isn't ultimately successful. A significant benefit of clinical research
is promoting generalizable knowledge that will improve practice for future
patients. But if the clinical community isn't persuaded by the research,
that benefit will never obtain. Wittes et al.'s (2007) discussion of the DSMB
deliberations for the Women's Health Initiative clinical trials illustrates this
point. Members of the DSMB were mindful of "the ambiguities that arose in
interpretation and in predicting the effect our recommendations would likely
have on the medical community" (Wittes et al. 2007, 219), aware that their
decisions sent messages to the medical community as a whole. According
to the DAMOCLES study group (2005, 714), "Statistical issues should be
only one of several considerations that a DMC needs to take into account.
Other considerations include the balance of primary risks and benefits, the
internal consistency of results, the consistency with, and nature of external
evidence, and the likelihood that the results would affect clinical practice."
While the goal of a trial should be to produce generalizable knowledge that
would "affect clinical practice," obtaining these data is a complex process.
Even when the DSMB, investigators, and sponsor are "entirely convinced,
(the study may require) continued randomization of participants to an inferior treatment regimen for the purpose of persuading practicing clinicians
whose openness to changing their practices may be very limited" (Ellenberg, Fleming, and DeMets 2019, 314).

E6 incorporates a notion of "indifference" between x and y, echoing
"lack of a grounded preference" in E2, distinct from E2's claim of "uncertainty." Once again, the patient's or research participant's preferences
are not taken into account—this lack of grounded preference captured by
"theoretical equipoise" or "clinical equipoise" is not the preference of those
actually taking x or y. DSMB members should be cautioned not to forget the
perspective of the research participant in all aspects of a trial's development
and execution.

With E7, we finally see patients' or participants' views explicitly addressed. Although it is still medical professionals who determine whether x and y are in equipoise, E7 makes explicit that equipoise is a step toward assuring patients and participants they will not be misused in a clinical trial. Given that "the acceptability of trial participation depends crucially on how the subject values the various probabilities and outcomes associated with trial enrollment" (Joffe and Truog 2008, 249), it is surprising that comparatively few notions of equipoise explicitly incorporate participants' views. Chapter 2's discussion of patient advocates raises the possibility of Joffe and Truog's fourth conception—equipoise as perceived among the community of potential participants and patients—being incorporated into study design after consultation with community advocates. Rather than equipoise being a determination of an individual physician or investigator (the first of Joffe and Truog's options, above), instead, it is the "professional community" that has not yet come to a consensus whether x or y is preferred (the third of Joffe and Truog's options). This was the case in AG and AH—although there were some clinicians using pneumonic vitreolysis, there was no consensus in the medical community whether this was in fact the best treatment to correct macular traction or to close a macular hole. Hence the need for protocols AG and AH, protocols designed to settle questions among clinicians as to whether pneumonic vitreolysis should be recommended. E7 claims the "professional community" needs to arrive at a consensus; even if the DSMB agrees about the relative virtues of x or y as study data rolls in, the evidence must be gathered and presented in such a way that the professional community would be convinced. For this reason, it is in the purview of DSMBs to review data quality and not just outcome data. Even if the DSMB is assured of the trial's equipoise, or that it has fallen out of equipoise, the DSMB must consider if the professional community will be similarly convinced. This echoes Freedman's concept of "clinical equipoise" that "an individual investigator or physician might have reasons to believe that one arm of the RCT offers therapeutic benefit over the other arm, but the medical profession as a whole remains divided" (Miller and Brody 2007, 203, citing Freedman). The concept of community equipoise is an important addition because it makes clear that clinical trials are part of a dialogue with professionals who may not be directly engaged in the trial.

Toward this end, some DSMBs are charged with reviewing and approving manuscripts that report the primary endpoints of the trial so as to ensure manuscripts reflect what actually happened in the trial, although this task is not explicitly mentioned in either the NIH's 1998 "Policy for Data Safety Monitoring" or the FDA's 2006 nonbinding "Guidance for Clinical Trial Sponsors." DeMets, Furberg, and Friedman (2006, 23) observe, "In many studies, even though the primary responsibility rests with the investigators, the monitoring committee is given the opportunity to review and comment on the draft manuscript for the main results and other major papers." The in-depth level of the engagement of the DSMB with the data, as well as their objective stance toward the research, afford the DSMB a position that is likely to be less biased than that of investigators. When DSMBs accept the responsibility to review and approve manuscripts this underscores the public nature of the research enterprise: the promotion of generalizable knowledge.

For this reason, a DSMB's recommendation to halt a trial early, if it appears to fall out of equipoise, is not merely a decision about protecting current research participants but also a decision about convincing members of the medical community of the wisdom of the DSMB's choice. In the case of protocols AG and AH, the persuasiveness of the evidence for stopping didn't end with the halting of the studies; the evidence needed to convince other practitioners not involved in the study to rethink broad use of pneumonic vitreolysis to treat macular traction or macular holes.

The DSMB can err by recommending that a trial be stopped too late, well after it has fallen out of equipoise, endangering participants by allowing a sponsor to needlessly keep them in a study arm in which they were harmed or denied benefit. The DSMB can also err by recommending that a trial be stopped too early. If the trial is stopped before sufficiently persuasive data are gathered, then the trial was not merely for naught; it was potentially harmful. The participants were exposed to the risks of the study without the benefit of new information being generated. Financial costs of the study were borne by the sponsors with nothing to show for that investment, although this concern is always secondary to the imperative to keep participants safe (DeMets, Furberg, and Friedman 2006). The complex calculus the DSMB undertakes, incorporating the interests of current participants, future patients, and the medical community as a whole, is about the weighing of beneficence and nonmaleficence obligations in overseeing clinical trials. When a DSMB recommends stopping a study early for falling out of equipoise the DSMB is advocating participants in the less efficacious arm not be harmed by occupying the arm into which they were randomized. Hence, stopping the trial may be a means of promoting non-maleficence for research participants. If a DSMB acts too quickly, and their recommendation that x and y are not in equipoise results in a stopped trial, but the trial's evidence fails to be persuasive to the professional community, the community may continue to believe that x and y are equally efficacious (Wittes et al. 2007). The result may be that the professional community continues prescribing x when they should have abandoned x for y. This then becomes a question of beneficence—a question of *preventing harm* as well as promoting good for future cohorts of patients who would have benefited from a definitive answer as to whether x or y should be preferred. One of the complexities of weighing off these obligations is that the violation of nonmaleficence, in harming current participants by retaining them in a study longer than necessary, is weighed against a possible violation of beneficence toward future as-yet-unidentified potential patients. Obligations of beneficence and nonmaleficence are difficult to weigh against each other in the most straightforward of circumstances. The DSMB is charged with weighing both obligations, as well as obligations to distinct cohorts. As Lantos and Feudtner (2015, 36) observe, "There is no completely objective way to determine whether a study ought or ought not to continue. If there were then there would be no need for DSMBs. Instead, there would be straightforward stopping rules that could be invoked by study statisticians whenever the predetermined statistical threshold was reached. Instead, DSMBs must make difficult judgment calls when interim analyses show worrisome trends that have not yet—or have just barely—reached statistical significance."

The complexities of the DSMB's responsibilities are magnified in light of the fact that the responses to equipoise determinations aren't always "all or nothing"; given the circumstances of each individual trial, the options for the DSMB may be more extensive than a black-and-white recommendation of stopping the study or continuing. The demand to maintain equipoise may necessitate a trial is *temporarily halted* until the DSMB can adequately sort out what appears to be happening, only to recommend resumption later. The DAMCOLES study group, noting the significance of these decisions, recommends that when a monitoring committee recommends stopping recruitment, they should do so in a meeting with the trial steering committee or sponsor. However, temporarily halting a trial comes with its own challenges. Temporarily halting recruitment may not be difficult as long as all sites can be promptly told to cease recruiting new participants. Some interventions may only be performed once, like the injection of gas in the AG and AH protocols. Follow-up to these interventions may continue, even if pausing the trial means no new participants are exposed to the experimental intervention. Other interventions may be logistically or clinically challenging to pause. The logistics of communicating to hundreds or thousands of participants in large phase III studies, for example, to temporarily stop taking a medication, and then recommending they subsequently can all resume, are daunting. Ellenberg, Fleming, and DeMets make the point that some larger trials may require more convincing statistical data for stopping (2019, 314). Some medications shouldn't be stopped overnight for fear of AEs; tapering dosage so that participants can safely halt taking medication adds additional layers of complexity. Recall the difficulties discussed in chapter 3 about "reconsenting" participants, including the logistical hurdles and the possibility that reconsenting will cause participants to lose faith in the study and withdraw, not to mention the debates among members of the DSMB as to whether the data truly indicate that "reconsent" is necessary. Many of the same issues emerge when considering whether to pause a study. The option to pause a trial may not be available for some studies, or in some cases, pausing would pose prohibitively difficult challenges, even if questions of equipoise do emerge.

Falling out of equipoise doesn't happen overnight. Even in cases in which SAEs are reported to the DSMB in an expedited manner, accumulating evidence that occupying arms x or y put participants at greater risk of harm, it may take weeks or months to amass sufficient statistical evidence that one arm is genuinely putting participants at greater risk. DSMBs may notice a worrying trend, but that trend may reverse itself before it reaches the level of a true signal that the study has fallen out of equipoise. In some cases, it isn't that the *entire trial* has fallen out of equipoise; rather, some subgroups may receive greater benefits, or be at a greater risk of harm, than others. In such a case, the DSMB may make recommendations that modify recruitment. In studies with more than two arms, it may be the case that one of the arms appears to present greater risk of harm or more than one arm shows evidence of benefit, but which of those beneficial arms is ultimately superior is unclear. In those cases, the DSMB may recommend to the sponsor that researchers *cease recruitment in some arms, but not in others.* As the complexity of the trial becomes greater—the increased number of participants, participants with varied inclusion criteria, a complex weighing-off of distinct benefits and risks that may result from participation, and compound or varied endpoints in the study—the more complex the assessment as to whether equipoise has been disrupted. The obligation to maintain equipoise involves intricate calculations about the nature of the statistical evidence, the unique experience of diverse participants, and the methodology employed in each study, mustering the expertise of statisticians, clinicians, and ethicists to keep participants safe.

Or so the arguments in favor of maintaining equipoise as a mainstay of DSMB work would have us think. The arguments in favor of protecting equipoise are complex. On the other side of the equipoise debate are several arguments in favor of abandoning equipoise as an ethical requirement in clinical trials. Two types of arguments in favor of maintaining equipoise are considered in this chapter. Arguments *against* maintaining equipoise are considered in chapter 6. Recall that equipoise emerges as an issue at two junctures in an RCT: Before a trial begins, it is expected to be in equipoise, and as the trial continues, it is supposed to remain in equipoise. Both of these claims will be considered.

Two Types of Arguments for Equipoise as Ethically Necessary

The bioethics literature is replete with arguments for and against the centrality of equipoise; an exhaustive presentation of either side would be prohibitive. However, the arguments in favor of equipoise can be grouped into two different sorts. The first are arguments that hold that *the very nature of the randomized controlled trial* presents an ethical justification for equipoise. The point of research is to gain knowledge that can help future patients. If that goal has already been achieved, it is a waste of resources such as participants, time, money, or professional expertise to reaffirm what is already known. That waste is itself ethically wrong, as researchers have a moral obligation to conserve the finite resources they are given to pursue scientific knowledge (Resnik 1998). London claims that in this way, equipoise, or lack thereof, "also provides the proper target for clinical research in that there is great social and clinical value in trials that are designed to disturb or to eliminate such a state of agnosticism or conflict" (London 2007a, 580). In keeping with Emanuel, Wendler, and Grady's (2000) claim that clinical research must be "socially valuable" (a claim further discussed in chapter 6), Borgerson (2016, 30) holds that "the social-value requirement exists partly to ensure that we are doing the best we can with the limited collective resources at our disposal, given our shared interest in advancing human health." This is why a study can, and should be, stopped per a DSMB's recommendation based on a finding of futility. Once it is recognized that no further effort in the trial will adequately address the primary endpoint, it is unethical to waste resources, including the time and potential health of participants. By the same token, if a study fails to be in equipoise at its inception—if it is *already known* that treatment option x is superior or inferior to treatment option y—the question driving the study had already been answered. This is one of the points that Wittes et al. (2007, 230) make about the Women's Health Initiative trials: "If anything, people were worried whether the hormone trials were ethical because the benefit on coronary disease, was, in their minds, so certain!"[4] Why squander the resources, including the risks of harm to research participants, if the question being asked has already been answered? If a study falls out of equipoise during its course—if treatment option x is shown definitively to be superior or inferior to treatment option y—what is the point in further engaging in the study? The reason for initiating the trial has been addressed.

Some might object to this argument by pointing to trials that replicate results of previous studies. Those studies use resources, including human participants. Surely those studies are of value, objectors may claim, especially in light of the so-called replication crisis in some areas of research (Hillary and Medaglia 2020; Hope et al. 2021). The replication crisis calls into question whether previous trials that *appeared* to have settled questions of generalizable knowledge have settled anything at all. Even when we think a research question is settled, there may be valid reasons to use resources to revisit those questions. Perhaps x was shown in a previous study to be superior, or inferior, to y, but after replication of the study, which supposedly settled the debate, it turns out that x's value isn't assured. Thus, the claim that a study isn't in equipoise may be an unconvincing reason not to commence the trial.

A reply to this objection recognizes that we do need to be careful, lest we go too far in declaring open season on all scientific claims, allowing any and all to be subject to replication. Not all clinical claims are created equal. Some claims of efficacy—on behalf of newer medications or techniques—may merit further study to demonstrate that initial claims can be replicated. Other long-standing claims—those with the backing of methodologically rigorous clinical trials or years of observational success—can, and should, be taken as fact so participants are not placed at risk of harm by needless replication of settled fact. Teasing out which of these claims are which isn't easy and requires the combined expertise of researchers, sponsors, research steering committees, medical monitors, granting agencies, and DSMB members. To dispute the centrality of equipoise, by claiming that it proves too much—namely, that it excludes the permissibility of replication studies—fails to take into account that not all scientific claims are supported by equally robust evidence. The protocol-specific expertise of the DSMB is one safeguard in ensuring that the clinical trial being proposed is not useless replication, but a valid use of valuable resources to address an open scientific question.

Note that this argument for the ethical centrality of equipoise based on the nature of clinical trials doesn't focus solely on the interests of research participants. One weakness of this argument is that it views research participants not as persons to be valued in themselves, but rather as resources that ought not be squandered. The argument doesn't rely on a duty of personal care, as Fried claimed, of researchers to their participants. For those who question if that duty of personal care exists, arguments based on the nature of clinical research may not be compelling.

For those who *do* hold that there is a duty of personal care in research, however, the duties of researchers, sponsors, and the DSMB, to keep people safe, present a second type of argument for the centrality of equipoise (Fried 1974). DSMBs are in place precisely because they are the body that has access to the entirety of data about the degree of harm and benefit to which participants are exposed while, at the same time, not directly interacting with participants. DSMBs review the data without bias and should not bias the outcome of the study by, for example, recommending changes in methodology or statistical analysis mid-study that puts the "thumb on the scale" of one or another arm. Thus, as they see the participants in one arm being harmed or being denied benefit in an arm by virtue of participation, it is the moral responsibility of the DSMB to advocate to prevent those harms or promote those benefits, not by changing methodology or analysis, but via other means. "The monitoring committee could recommend stopping the study (or, in the case of a multi-armed study, dropping one arm) for any of several reasons. These include such overwhelming evidence of benefit from the intervention that the study hypothesis was answered earlier than expected or sufficient evidence of unexpected serious harm" (DeMets, Furberg, and Friedman 2006, 10).

This argument is an argument about moral duties owed to participants: Beneficence and nonmaleficence toward participants demand that they aren't unduly denied benefit, or harmed, by virtue of their enrollment in an RCT. Even if they have offered autonomous consent, participants are owed the moral protections afforded by equipoise. Defenders of this position don't make the claim that equipoise is sufficient for ethical research, only necessary. Other provisions, such as informed consent, or non-exploitation, may also be necessary for research to be ethical, but equipoise is required. Protecting equipoise is what allows a participant to, in good faith, enroll in what Jerry Menikoff and Edward P. Richards (2006) call "bad choice studies"—studies in which a participant may not personally benefit, or may even experience risks of harm, but the expectation is that future cohorts may benefit from the knowledge gained. The participant in a bad choice study may recognize the unlikely personal benefit from study enrollment. But to be used as a participant in a study initiated by investigators who know that the scales are balanced against participants from the start, or to be used in a study that is sustained even after it is established which arm definitively produces greater harms or greater benefits, is an ethical lapse on the part of the researchers. Participants who enroll in "good choice studies," in which they are expected to benefit directly from the research, are being treated with beneficence. Those who enroll in "bad choice studies" are at least owed the fact that the study is done in good faith for the benefit of others, even if they aren't expected to benefit themselves. Freedman's distinction between "theoretical equipoise" and "clinical equipoise" was conceived to allow him to maintain the duties of personal care of a treating physician, even against a backdrop of conflicting professional views about the merits of competing treatments. Hence, an ethical study could be in equipoise, even if the treating physician had personal preferences about the merits of one arm of the study over another. The duties of personal care to research participants, to not be treated merely as a means (Hellman and Hellman 1991), make clear the ethical requirements of researchers and those who guide them.

Equipoise and Protocols AG and AH

Protocols AG and AH enrolled forty-six and thirty-five participants, respectively. Protocol AG was a placebo-controlled RCT, in which the participants were masked as to whether they received the gas injection or a placebo, a sham "injection."[5] The sham injections weren't injections of a different gas than perfluoropropane; the sham consisted of participants being *told* they were being given a gas injection, but receiving nothing at all. Protocol AH wasn't a randomized controlled trial—there was a single arm in which all participants received gas injections. Both studies were believed to be in equipoise by the researchers, sponsor, IRB, and DSMB when they commenced. Patients who experience macular traction or a macular hole can lose a significant vision. While both macular traction and macular holes correct on their own in about 30 percent of cases, this process isn't guaranteed and can take a long time. The injection of gas to correct macular traction or a macular hole had previously been used by some practitioners and had been reported on in the medical literature; injection of gas to correct macular traction/holes wasn't entirely novel. Published studies indicated that the gas injections might be promising to correct macular traction or holes. As such, there were compelling reasons to believe the benefits of the injections might outweigh the risks—risks such as the traction/hole never correcting, or correcting only after an extended period of time. The most common treatment for closing a macular hole is a surgery called vitrectomy. Vitrectomy comes with its own risks, such as the progression of cataracts, and in rare cases, a significant and potentially vision-endangering infection, endophthalmitis. It was up to the discretion of the participant's treating ophthalmologist if the patient needed vitrectomy during the course of the study—surgery was not ruled out for patients in either study. For this reason, the risks of protocols AG and AH didn't include being denied further treatment; rescue surgery, if indicated, was not considered a protocol deviation. Silverman and Dreyfuss (2014) observe that if a trial doesn't allow flexibility of practitioner discretion over the course of the protocol, the study might result in a "less favorable risk-benefit profile." Such a lack of flexibility might lead to greater "net risks" for those in the experimental arms, in keeping with the "net risks" test proposed by Wendler and Miller in chapter 3. This was not a concern in protocols AG and AH, fortunately.

Rather, the point of the gas injections was to see *if surgery could be initially avoided*, but not precluded altogether.

Although there were potential benefits to receiving the injections, such as the traction/hole resolving without surgery, the injections could come with unknown risks. Taking all the above into account, the study designs—in which the participants were randomized into either a gas injection or placebo (AG) or solely given the gas injections (AH), then watched carefully to see if the traction/holes resolved, with local practitioners permitted to use their best judgment if surgery was warranted—were found to be in equipoise.

> After 62 participants enrolled in the two studies, the DSMC noted the rate of retinal tear or detachment was more than the estimate in the informed consent form (1%). . . . The DSMC recommended suspension of enrollment and for the study group to review these cases, to inform investigators, and to revise the informed consent form. The informed consent form and protocol were revised to include a retinal detachment incidence range of 5% to 13%. . . . After resumption of enrollment, additional retinal tears and detachments occurred, bringing the combined total from both studies to 7 of the 59 eyes that received the gas injection (12%; 95% CI, 6%–23%), and the DSMC recommended termination of recruitment. (Chan et al. 2021, 1600–1601)

At the time recruitment was halted, 46 of the target 124 participants in AG had been enrolled, and all 35 of the participants in AH had been enrolled. The studies ran for fifteen months, during which 12 percent of the participants who received the gas injection experienced either a retinal tear or a retinal detachment.[6] Some of those who experienced the retinal tear or retinal detachment could have lost considerable vision from those SAEs. Further adding to the risk profile was the fact that some participants' vision wasn't initially poor—the inclusion criteria for participants included having vision that was the equivalent of between 20/32 and 20/400 in AG, with the mean visual acuity being 20/50 in the treatment group and 20/40 in the sham group. In AH, the inclusion criteria included a visual acuity of between 20/25 and 20/400, with a mean of 20/80 (Chan et al. 2021, 1595). 20/400 is significantly compromised vision, but at 20/40 vision is not that compromised.[7] In sum, participants who may not have had poor vision upon enrollment in the study were placed at risk of retinal tears or retinal detachment that was higher than initially expected, thereby compromising the balance of potential benefits over possible risks of the study.

A monitoring committee's decision to act when a trial risks falling out of equipoise—to recommend temporary suspension of recruitment pending more information, to recommend halting recruitment in one arm, or to recommend stopping a trial altogether—isn't always based on data that is unambiguous or that appears overnight or on a once-every-six-month pre-established meeting schedule. The process of tipping out of equipoise may be protracted, and the decision to recommend temporarily halting a study, modifying arms, or stopping the study altogether may not be unanimously endorsed by the entire committee. In the case of AG and AH, the committee first recommended halting recruitment in light of the unexpected increase in SAEs and then recommended resumption of the protocol with modification of informed consent that altered participants to adjusted probabilities of SAEs. Modifications of informed consent in the midst of a study, as discussed in chapter 3, come with their own complexities. Despite the need for a revision of the informed consent, the data had not yet convinced the monitoring committee that the study had fallen out of equipoise.

After the study resumed, however, reports of continued retinal tears and retinal detachments persisted. In AG, there were no tears or detachments in the sham group—all occurred in participants who received the experimental gas injections. These SAEs were considerable enough that in the committee's view the studies fell out of equipoise. They recommended stopping both studies. AG falling out of equipoise was about the sham arm conferring fewer risks than the treatment arm. In AH, the recruitment goal had been reached, so there was a sense in which the study wasn't stopped on the basis of the committee's recommendation. There was no way to "undo" the injection of the gas into the eyes of the AH participants. It was fortunate that no additional participants were put at risk.

A final note about the discussion of AG and AH: The above discussion is but one example of a monitoring committee I served on, although I've served on many. Although I framed my discussion around these two trials, this discussion is not meant to be representative of every equipoise debate. As pointed out earlier, disputes about a study's equipoise may reflect the complexity of the study itself. Studies that involve a greater number of participants, participants with diverse inclusion criteria, complex endpoints, and that appear to be yielding complex data about a combination of benefits and risks, are even more fraught when it comes to determinations of equipoise (DeMets and Ellenberg 2016). The back-and-forth among the members of the data monitoring committee, the sponsor, and the data coordinating center for the AG and AH trials, as reported by the publicly disclosed discussion, involved recommendations to initially start the trial, suspend the trial, resume the trial after altering the informed consent, and finally terminate the trial. Now imagine increasing the AG and AH protocols, which collectively enrolled fewer than one hundred participants, to the size of some phase III trials that recruit hundreds, or even thousands, of participants. The difficulty in preserving equipoise becomes even more challenging.

Conclusion

One of the most consequential responsibilities of DSMBs is to review studies to ensure that they are in equipoise before they begin and to review data as it accumulates so as to ensure that studies remain in equipoise. The sponsor, researchers, and IRB all have a role alongside the DSMB to ensure that studies commence in equipoise, but because the DSMB has access to the entirety of the study data as it comes in, they are in a privileged position when it comes to assessing the continued equipoise of any trial. There are competing analyses of what the term *equipoise* means and distinct types of arguments in favor of the centrality of equipoise. Examining these competing analyses, as well as arguments in favor of maintaining equipoise, helps to clarify the scope and importance of a DSMB's charge. As data accumulates, the DSMB may be asked to weigh in on an emergency basis. New findings, or expedited reports of SAEs, don't arrive on a fixed schedule. Those who agree to serve on a DSMB must be willing to dedicate extensive time to review materials in advance of meetings, to engage other members in analysis of complex data, and to be available to respond to urgent calls for hastily convened meetings to address unexpected issues (Herson 2017, 28). For research participants in AG or AH who experienced a retinal tear or retinal detachment, that AE can reasonably be assumed to be *one of the most important events in their lives* at the time it occurred. Members of DSMBs should recognize the gravity of each participant's sacrifice in volunteering for a clinical trial and take up their charge with the requisite sense of responsibility. DSMB members need to take seriously their duties to participants, including potentially recommending a stop to research when its risks outweigh its benefits. Expedited reporting of SAEs may necessitate changes to a consent form in the middle of a study. Data trends may demonstrate that a study's ability to answer a question is futile or that a study has fallen out of equipoise, in which case it is unethical to continue. Finally, there may be struggles with recruitment, or an unexpected event such as COVID, which require extensive work with study sponsors to keep projects moving, while at the same time keeping participants safe. These last challenges are the subject of the next chapter.

5 Recruitment, Retention, and Keeping Vulnerable Participants Safe: The SIGHT Trial

Idiopathic intercranial hypertension (IIH) can lead to progressive vision loss by narrowing the range of an individual's visual field.[1] For example, a patient can start with a visual field that ranges 160 degrees from side to side but erodes down to low double digits. This narrowing of a visual field is debilitating. There are several treatment strategies available, but it is unclear which of these is the most effective. The SIGHT trial (Surgical Intercranial Hypertension Treatment trial; official title "Randomized Trial of Medical Therapy (MT) vs. MT Plus Optic Nerve Sheath Fenestration vs. MT Plus Ventriculoperitoneal Cerebrospinal Fluid Shunting in Subjects with Idiopathic Intercranial Hypertension and Moderate to Severe Visual Loss") was a phase III study designed to recruit 180 patients with IIH and vision loss. Participants would be randomized to one of three arms to examine which arm best treated visual field loss. The first arm was medical (drug) therapy, a diuretic plus weight management counseling. The second treatment arm was the diuretic, weight management counseling, and a surgery called optic nerve sheath fenestration (ONSF), designed to release the tension on the optic nerve that may be contributing to vision loss. The third arm included the diuretic, weight management counseling, and surgery called ventriculoperitoneal CSF shunting (VPS). VPS involves placing a shunt catheter in the skull that drains fluid into the abdomen, thereby relieving the intercranial pressure. Participants would be evaluated for the primary outcome, a measure of visual field, at six months, and they would be followed for an additional three years. If the patients didn't meet the primary outcome at six months, they would be eligible for a new treatment based on their physician's recommendation. SIGHT was terminated after sixteen participants were recruited during a two-year period.[2]

Barriers to Recruitment I: Connecting to Marginalized Participants

There is no single answer why the SIGHT trial was unable to successfully recruit participants. The trial included many strengths. The PIs and local investigators were extremely well qualified and passionate about the trial.

The sponsor—the NEI—was similarly enthusiastic. The rationale for the study—determining which of three treatments was the best way to address vision loss due to IIH—was and remains a much-needed public health imperative. The data-coordinating center was top-notch, and I was honored to serve on its DSMB, which comprised some of the leading lights in the field.

The DSMB met with the investigators twice annually during the two years that SIGHT was active. Recruitment of participants became an early concern. Lagging recruitment at the two-year mark was not a bolt from the blue. Nonetheless, when SIGHT was terminated, it was a significant disappointment to the researchers, the NEI, the DSMB, and the participants who had been recruited and randomized. Although some participants may have been expected to directly benefit from participation, receiving a treatment for IIH that was superior to the treatment in the other arms this was not guaranteed. Rather, the primary benefit of the study was learning which of the three treatment arms was most successful for future IIH patients. The enrolled and randomized SIGHT participants experienced the risks of their respective treatment arms without any of the benefit of generalized knowledge from the SIGHT trial's completion. For that reason, it was ethically fraught for the DSMB to terminate the SIGHT study. Wertheimer argues that prospective subjects be told if a study may prematurely end because of low enrollment (Wertheimer 2014), precisely because it *is* an ethical lapse when research participants are exposed to risks of trials that do not reap the benefits of generalizable knowledge. Like much information conveyed as part of informed consent—the risks of experimental treatments, the potential costs in terms of money and time, and the potential for violations of confidentiality—telling participants that trials can prematurely end because of low enrollment may jeopardize enrollment in a study or cause participants additional anxiety during the already fraught experience of participating in research. However, if Wertheimer is correct, this is information that participants should know so that their decision to enroll is well informed. Participants are routinely told if there is a risk that they can be removed from a study, perhaps owing to a determination by their local doctor, a funding issue, or a determination by an oversight body such as the IRB or DSMB. Telling potential participants of yet another way in which the study could fail, while potentially causing additional concern, may be a necessary part of fully informing participants of what enrollment might entail.

Unfortunately, the SIGHT DSMB didn't see a clear path to the timely recruitment of 180 participants, a number required to demonstrate with sufficient statistical power which of the three arms was superior, given that only sixteen participants had been recruited over two years. "Clinical trials, indeed all clinical research, are only ethical if there is a reasonable expectation that important information will result, i.e., that clinically meaningful questions can be answered. If, during the course of a trial, it becomes clear that no such outcome is likely, the study may be stopped for what has been termed 'futility'" (DeMets, Furberg, and Friedman 2006, 22). "The DSMB also may determine that a trial should be stopped if lack of adherence to the protocol or poor enrollment makes it unlikely that the objectives of the trial will be met" (Gordon, Sugarman, and Kass 1998, 2). Without being able to recruit sufficient participants, the SIGHT trial was unable to assess which of the three arms was preferable for treating IIH. Although it was a difficult decision for the DSMB to recommend stopping the trial, it was the ethically right call.

DSMBs spend a significant amount of time monitoring recruitment and retention. The potential benefits of a trial are only possible if the trials meet their recruitment goals, and meet them in a timely fashion. Here, DSMB recommendations can run the gamut from enthusiastic cheerleading, to anxious concern, to scolding warning of researcher efforts. When recruitment or retention lags, or dropouts are high, DSMBs may be consulted about revision of recruitment strategies, study procedures, or statistical analysis so that some benefits of the study can be retained in the face of these challenges. Some considerations are more fraught than others. Since the DSMB has access to unblinded data that the researchers may not, the DSMB needs to be cautious when endorsing a change to the statistical analysis plan that would affect study conclusions. As discussed previously, Wittes et al. (2007) stressed that any requests made by the DSMB during the course of the study may telegraph to the researchers information about the study to which they are blinded, thereby potentially creating bias.

Monitoring recruitment is akin to other activities of DSMBs reviewed in chapter 1, which, on their face, may not appear directly implicated in patient safety but are nonetheless essential. Responsible study conduct, including recruitment and data management, is part of DSMB oversight. According to the FDA's "Guidance for Clinical Trial Sponsors" (2006, 20),

"The DMC typically shares responsibility for assessment of data related to study conduct with the sponsor, the study leadership (such as a steering committee) and to some extend with IRBs." DSMBs have a role in monitoring protocol deviations that compromise data integrity. According to the European Medicines Agency (2005, 5), "If major problems with the study conduct are observed, a DMC should consider possible recommendations to the sponsor to improve the quality of the study." DSMBs may receive reports as to whether qualified personnel are collecting data, as well as information as to whether data analysis is being done accurately, timely, and consistently. They have a role in recommending to sponsors or steering committees changes to study procedures to maintain data integrity.

I've seen a lot of hand-wringing over low recruitment, low retention, and high dropout rates, and the ways in which studies may be in jeopardy owing to those concerns. Collins (2003, 71) recounts the experience of one monitoring board when faced with low recruitment: "The DSMB recommended placing the study on probation and replacing poorly performing sites. At their second annual meeting, the DSMB recommended approval of proposed changes to the study design contingent on the study leadership removing nonproductive sites. These changes were a 2-year increase in the recruitment period and a change in study design that decreased required sample size. Nonproductive centers were terminated and the approved changes allowed the study to be successfully completed."

The above actions by the DSMB—removing unproductive sites, reducing sample size, which would allow for the prospective benefits of the study to obtain—are well within the purview of the DSMB. Making these changes doesn't come without costs. There is significant time and expense onboarding new sites to replace those lagging in recruitment. Not having a large enough sample may compromise the ability to do all analyses researchers had initially planned. The DSMB is responsible for weighing these costs against the costs of not completing the research in a timely manner, or perhaps not at all, owing to slow recruitment.

I like to think DSMBs could anticipate barriers to recruitment before they occur, offering recommendations to researchers to avoid recruit challenges and the costs of addressing them mid-study. According to the DAMOCLES study group (2005, 712), "The potential roles for a DMC before trial recruitment starts have received little attention in published work." There are two factors that may have played a part in the low recruitment in SIGHT. Both are considerations the researchers and DSMB could have anticipated and possibly addressed proactively. The first concerns the research participants themselves. The second concerns the study's methodology.

Understanding the barriers to recruitment in the SIGHT study first requires an understanding of the intersectional biases that confronted SIGHT's participants. According to Wall (2017, 45), "Idiopathic intracranial hypertension (IIH) is a disorder of overweight women in the childbearing age characterized by increased intracranial pressure with its associated signs and symptoms in an alert and oriented patient." Elsewhere, IIH is said to "primarily affect(s) obese women" (Boyter 2019, 30). IIH "most often occurs in obese women of childbearing age . . . the annual incidence of idiopathic intercranial hypertension is increasing in association with obesity rates" (Thurtell 2019, 1289).

One of the reasons the SIGHT trial was important was that it investigated treatments for a medical condition that primarily affects women, a population that historically has been under-investigated. In 1993, the FDA instituted that both men and women be studied in clinical trials and that women of child-bearing potential could not be systemically excluded from clinical trials. The NIH was similarly directed by Congress to ensure that women, as well as members of minority groups, were proactively included in government-sponsored studies (Dresser 2008, 235). Dresser argues that the principles of beneficence in promoting good for current and future patient populations, autonomy in promoting freedom of choice, and justice in promoting equal access, all support moves toward expanded access to participation in clinical trials (Dresser 2008, 235–236). However, expanded access can also bring further burdens of serving in research, or the possibility of enrollment under misinformed or exploitive circumstances.

Although greater inclusion of women in research studies is a net positive, it is also the case that gender discrimination in health care is well documented. SteelFisher et al. (2019) surveyed a nationally representative sample of 1,596 women, finding that 18 percent of women in the United States experienced discrimination in health care. Eighteen percent may seem like a comparatively low number (less than a fifth!), but surely any amount of discrimination in health care is too high. Since IIH patients are most likely to be women, the expectation is that many of them previously experienced discrimination in the health-care system.

According to the Urban Institute, "More than 4 in 10 adults in the US are affected by obesity" (Urban Institute 2022). Persons with obesity experience

well-documented discrimination in health care. Phelan et al. (2015) summarize their findings in a review that examined all articles in two databases,
PubMed and PsychInfo, on obesity stigma in health care published prior to
fall 2014. They summarize (2014, 319): "Many healthcare providers hold
strong negative attitudes and stereotypes about people with obesity. There
is considerable evidence that such attitudes influence person-perceptions,
judgment, interpersonal behaviour and decision-making. These attitudes
may impact the care they provide. Experiences of or expectations for poor
treatment may cause stress and avoidance of care, mistrust of doctors and
poor adherence among patients with obesity. Stigma can reduce the quality
of care for patients with obesity despite the best intentions of healthcare
providers to provide high-quality care." IIH patients are likely to be persons
with obesity whose health care, and whose expectations of health care,
has been marred by discrimination, lack of trust, and systemic inability to
adhere to a program of care. The participants in the SIGHT study may have
already experienced discrimination in the health-care system by virtue of
gender or obesity. Thus, the potential SIGHT participants may have had
two reasons to expect bias in their interactions with the SIGHT investigators. However, the basis for their expectations of bias and discrimination
may have had even more extensive roots.

According to the Urban Institute (2022, 1), "Black, Hispanic/Lantinx,
Native American and Alaskan Native, and Pacific Islander communities
experience higher rates of obesity than white and Asian adults. Awareness
of these disparities and their root causes provides important context for
assessing place-based differences and for understanding how averages can
also mask important differences within communities." The Urban Institute's data demonstrate a significant gap between the rates of obesity in
Black and white populations, and Lantinx and white populations, including in state-by-state comparisons. SteelFisher et al. also found the rates
of discrimination in health care for both Black and Latinx respondents is
far higher than their white counterparts. As Linda Villarosa has carefully
documented, a history of racial bias, both overt and systemic, has plagued
the medical profession (Villarosa 2022). The result is both consistently
poorer health outcomes in minority communities and a well-earned wari-
ness among members of minority communities of health-care professionals. "Mistrust seems to be significantly higher in minority populations than

among whites, and it can affect the type of medical care that members of minority populations seek and receive" (Specker Sullivan 2020, 20).

Studies have found that there is a negative correlation between socio-economic status and obesity in the United States (Sobal and Stunkard 1989; Metha and Chang 2009). It is possible that having fewer resources means fewer, and less healthy, food options, in which case, lower socioeconomic status may contribute to obesity. The relationship between obesity and income is a complex one; at least one study has postulated that owing to discrimination, in both the labor market and social stigmatization, persons with obesity end up in lower-paying jobs than those who are not obese (Kim and Knesebeck 2018). In other words, it isn't clear if lower socioeconomic status causes obesity, owing to having less money for healthy foods or being unable to access transportation away from food deserts that restrict choices, or if obesity causes lower socioeconomic status, owing to discrimination in the labor market. Irrespective of the causal relationship, obesity is correlated with lower socioeconomic status.

Thus, the participants in the SIGHT study were more likely to be women, more likely to be persons discriminated against because of obesity, more likely to be members of minority communities, and more likely to be of a lower socioeconomic status. Possibly all four could be true. By contrast, researchers "tend to be relatively healthy, well educated, and affluent. As a result, research professionals might not experience the same pressures, risks, burdens and inconveniences as other subjects" (Dresser 2017, 38). Unlike many of the researchers and members of the DSMB, potential SIGHT participants were likely to be from historically marginalized communities ill-treated by the medical profession. The mistaken belief that the participants are similar to researchers is an example of what John Lynch calls "researcher ethnocentrism" (Lynch 2011). Falling into mistaken assumptions informed by researcher ethnocentrism can result in a failure to meet participants where they are with respect to values, preferences, or even quotidian considerations such as the opportunity cost of leaving work early for yet another medical exam. The researchers and DSMB should have been sensitive to the complexities of recruiting participants with intersectional identities in the SIGHT study.

The benefits of the SIGHT trial to members of historically marginalized communities were extensive—losing vision is a significant impairment. If visual impairment results from a condition correlated with obesity, this may continue to be a mounting problem in the United States. Researchers who study IIH are an impressive lot by virtue of their commitment to a disease that affects marginalized communities that don't often garner headlnes. Advocates "suspect that scientists have been overly responsive to certain interest groups" (Dresser 2008, 236; Largent, Fernandez Lynch, and McCoy 2018), but younger women, the obese, or members of other marginalized communities aren't typically among those privileged groups.

Even though the public health implications of the SIGHT trial were vast, the hurdles to recruiting members of the IIH population were also vast. Whether or not those potential participants had a right to be suspicious of the researchers in the SIGHT trial is beside the point. *The researchers* had good reason to think that their potential participants would be wary and were in a position to proactively address those concerns. Bioethicists who study research ethics are familiar with the concepts of therapeutic misconception, "the mistaken belief that decisions about one's treatment while a research subject would be made solely based on one's individual condiion and needs" (Appelbaum and Lidz 2008, 633); therapeutic misestimation, in which a "research subject underestimates risk, overestimates benefi, or both" (Horng and Grady 2003 11); unrealistic optimism (Jansen et al. 2011), and similar cognitive biases promoting participation under false pretenses (Swekoski and Barnbaum 2013). Therapeutic misconception or unrealistic optimism can lead patients to enroll in research studies thinking they will receive direct benefits or they will not end up in the placebo group. Dresser (2017) speaks of participants whose trust and faith in the medical profession may cause them to mistakenly believe that trial enrollment and randomization, for example, will be tailored to be of direct benefit. Bioethicists must also take seriously the flip side of that coin: potential participants whose *lack of faith and trust in the medical profession might prevent them from enrolling* or position them as ready to withdraw from a study at the drop of a hat. The DSMB had a significant role in addressing and anticipating these concerns, pressing the researchers to ensure their means of recruitment and retention were tailored to address these issues. Metcalfe and Park (2024) advocate that risk-based monitoring include monitoring of the diversity action plan researchers put in place to ensure that recruited participants are diverse. The DSMB may have a role in both monitoring diversity action plans and helping to shape them so as to ensure compliance with FDA mandates.

Setting aside the intersectional biases that may have confronted the SIGHT study participants, there may be something about the very nature of enrolling in a clinical trial that deters potential participants. Participants may be wary owing to historical injustices in which people were enrolled without consent or mistreated in clinical trials. Reluctance may be based on something as mundane, however, as health information being collected and tracked, which some may view as a violation of privacy. Dresser calls attempts to maintain compliance with research methodology, such as monitors to check for pill consumption or exercise tracking, "policing"; such strategies often "reinforce the research hierarchy" in which participants are on the bottom and researchers are on top (Dresser 2017, 107). All three arms of the SIGHT study involved "medical management," in which participants were required to take medication to reduce their weight, as well as weight loss counseling. Pills would be tracked, counselors would remind people what to eat and what not to, and participants would be weighed. Whether or not the term "policing" came up in any discussion among potential SIGHT participants, the sentiment may have been enough to drive some participants away. For this reason, Dresser advocates a more collaborative approach, in which former and potential research participants are more actively engaged in the structure and oversight of research (Dresser 2008). Recruitment by individuals who are not necessarily affiliated with the research project, but who come from communities that the participant population trusts, can be integrated into the protocol (Appelbaum and Lidz 2008). Some hurdles to greater inclusion of women, minorities, and other marginalized groups can be traversed: "Barriers to fully inclusive trials do exist but are surmountable with investment and focused, sustained, community-partnered effort" (Bibbins-Domingo, Helman, and Dzau 2022). The model discussed in chapter 2, in which DSMBs include both an ethicist and a patient advocate, might have been particularly helpful in the SIGHT trial. A patient advocate from the IIH community may have been able to speak to some of the issues surrounding bias in health care or the perception that research interventions and data collection were at risk of seemingly "policing" participants, thereby hindering recruitment.

DSMBs consider issues pursuant to keeping participants safe: informed consent, establishing that the potential benefits of the study outweigh the potential risks at the onset, and ensuring that the study doesn't fall out of equipoise. In addition to these, it is also within the purview of the DSMB to examine accrual, recruitment, and retention issues even though recruitment and retention may not immediately seem to be about keeping participants safe. The NIH's 1998 "Policy for Data and Safety Monitoring" explicitly states that "recruitment, accrual and retention" are within the purview of monitoring committees. Recruitment is one of the most challenging bottlenecks to the completion of successful research: "A shortfall of participants in biomedical research impedes clinical trials more than a lack of funding" (Schaefer, Emanuel, and Wertheimer 2009, 70), a concern that has resulted for some to call for fewer clinical trials (Borgerson 2016).

One way of demonstrating that successful recruitment and retention *are* related to safety considers an analogy between data collection and statistical analysis on one hand, and recruitment and retention strategies on the other. No DSMB would have voted to approve a study if the data collection or statistical analysis plans were inadequate, because these inadequacies would have yielded a study that exposed participants to all the risks of the trial, without yielding the benefits of generalizable results. In the same vein, studies that have ill-defined recruitment and retention plans hazard exposing participants to the possible risks of the trial, while never producing the potential benefit of generalizable results. Recruitment and retention *are* issues of benefit and risk, and insofar as they are issues of benefit and risk, they are an issue of participant safety. DSMBs have a role in monitoring both adherence to study procedures, so as to ensure the integrity of the data, and recruitment, retention, and dropout rates to determine the study will be completed. The DSMB in SIGHT was positioned to advocate more strongly for a recruitment and retention plan that would have promoted a better balance of potential benefits over risks.

With the benefit of hindsight, knowing what happened in the SIGHT trial, what more could have been done? Other recommendations have been offered, in addition to the inclusion of a patient advocate on the DSMB. Angus, Gordon, and Bauchner (2021), as well as Blumenthal and James (2022), though not discussing SIGHT specifically, argue there should be greater coordination nationally to recruit potential participants. As things currently stand, each set of local investigators is on its own, trying to recruit for individual studies while at the same time competing against duties of clinical care for the patients, but also competing against other clinical trials. This competition may put local researchers in a bind, as they are asked to recruit for multiple clinical trials that are drawing from the same subject pool (Barnbaum 2019). When sponsors seek enrollment from minority communities, but this enrollment is lagging, Herson says it is within the purview of monitoring committees to recommend sponsors appoint an enrollment "czar" who can coordinate efforts toward more diverse enrollment (Herson 2017, 57). The DSMB could have pressed researchers for a more complete plan to recruit participants, including forming networks with other researchers and community-based organizations. No researcher can build from scratch the kind of nationally coordinated model Angus, Gordon, and Bauchner argue for. Still, a smaller-scale plan might have made a difference.

Barriers to Recruitment II: Study Methodology

A second obstacle to recruitment in the SIGHT trial may have been the randomization scheme. Participants in SIGHT would be randomized to either 1) medical management (medication) and weight loss counseling, 2) medical management, weight loss counseling, plus one type of surgery (ONSF), or 3) medical management, weight loss counseling, plus a different type of surgery (VPS). The SIGHT trial was a *randomized* controlled trial—once participants agreed to be in the study, they had no say as to which of the three treatments they would receive. Randomization is so common it is reasonable to assume that randomization alone hasn't undermined most trials. The studies discussed in chapters 2–4 were all initiated as RCTs. Despite the fact that the CALEC study changed course from its initial conception, CALEC, SIGHT-IPF, and protocols AG and AH did not encounter the hurdles that befell SIGHT. What may have set SIGHT apart was not randomization alone, but randomization among a particular set of treatment arms. Without getting into the specifics of the risk profile, invasiveness, recovery time, or follow-up schedule of ONSF versus VPS, it is reasonable to assume some participants may have preferred one type of surgery over the other or preferred the drug-only option over surgery, or vice versa. Recall that the initial design of the CALEC study discussed in chapter 2 was between two different surgeries (CALEC and CLAU), which were fairly similar. The arms in SIGHT, however, included two radically different surgeries or the option of not having surgery at all. While the clinical community may have viewed the three SIGHT arms to be in equipoise, each potential participant may have had strong reasons to prefer one arm over the other. Those preferences can affect a participant's willingness to be randomized. In their review of empirical literature on randomization, Joffe and Truog (2008) found physicians and prospective participants often have preferences among arms in studies. The perception that studies aren't in equipoise on the part of local investigators, and significantly *potential participants*, may undercut recruitment. Open-label studies that randomize standard-of-care drugs against what participants may view as potentially life-saving new therapies can lag in recruitment for this very reason. Participants may enroll, find that they have been randomized to standard-of-care, and subsequently drop out, as they had preferred the new therapy.[3] Here the lessons from the earlier discussion of equipoise emerge. Joffe and Truog (2008, 249) previously observed "the acceptability of trial participation depends crucially on how the subject values the various probabilities and outcomes associated with trial enrollment." Incorporating patient preferences, per suggestions by Floyd and Moyer (2010) or Janevic et al. (2003), may have promoted recruitment. "Even in the absence of agreement in the medical community regarding general preferences for treatment of a given condition, there may be important reasons to favor one over another for particular patients" (Appelbaum and Lidz 2008, 634). If patients were able to enroll in SIGHT choosing their preferred arm, rather than be subject to randomization perhaps recruitment would have been more successful.

It may be argued that by the time a study is reviewed by DSMB, but before the study begins to recruit participants, it is too late to change aspects of the methodology, such as whether the study is randomized. This point may be persuasive; however, an objection to this claim considers all the aspects of the study about which DSMB *does* offer recommendations. Both before and during the course of a study the DSMB may end up recommending changes to the statistical analysis plan, the consent form, the recruitment strategy, and the type of data that is collected. As pointed out in chapter 4, the FDA says data monitoring committees may recommend changing eligibility criteria, altering dosage levels, and altering recruitment criteria (U.S. Department of Health and Human Services 2006, 19). There are limits to what the DSMB can responsibly recommend; for example, recommending changes to a statistical analysis plan after the DSMB had seen critical interim data, or requesting additional data collection that negatively affected the balance of benefits over risks, would be unacceptable. However, given the extensive reach the DSMB has, it makes sense it would have some say about methodology before a study begins, including whether the study is randomized.

Some researchers might argue the only way to know which of these three treatments was best for the vision-affecting IIH was to perform an RCT; without randomization, study results would have been compromised. The open-label studies mentioned above, which are unable to recruit because participants simply drop out if they aren't randomized into their preferred arm are a cautionary tale. The studies may also be compromised in that even if they are able to meet their accrual goals, the data may be suspect. This is a compelling point; RCTs are considered the gold standard of research methodologies, with unrandomized studies perceived as less persuasive. Furthermore, it isn't merely *the researchers* who need to be convinced of the superiority, or inferiority, or one arm over the others—as seen in chapter 4, it is *the entire clinical community* that needs to be convinced. In response to this argument one might ask, What profits a researcher, or the clinical community, if the preferred methodology is maintained, only to have the study fail for lack of recruitment? The orthodoxy that RCTs are the gold standard of clinical methodologies is firmly entrenched, but perhaps too firmly entrenched across the board for the goals of research and the promotion of health. It may be incumbent upon the DSMB to question whether the researcher team's preferred methodology is also the most ethical way of conducting a study. One thing is clear, as illustrated by the SIGHT trial: A failed RCT does no one any good, whether the researchers, future patients, or the current participants whose time and effort come to naught. If the benefits of generalizable knowledge could be achieved via some other methodology than the traditional randomized controlled trial, that alternative methodology would have been worth pursuing. If there is no alternative methodology that would have yielded the benefits of generalizable knowledge, then perhaps it is better that no trial take place than one that exposes participants to risks without any potential benefit.

Joffe and Truog (2008) endorse options laid out by Veatch (1987) and Silverman (1994), advocating "semi-randomized" or "comprehensive cohort" trials. In these studies, participants are offered the choice of different arms; participants could choose a given arm or choose randomization. Conceivably, SIGHT participants who were so empowered may have been more likely to remain in the study. Even those who didn't have a preference among arms may nonetheless have appreciated exercising their autonomy to make a selection. Affording potential participants autonomy can demonstrate respect for participants, so that even if they end up relinquishing some choice, they feel valued as people. In semi-randomized trials, the primary endpoint would consider only data from those who agreed to randomization. Joffe and Truog maintain that data from the participants who chose their assignment would nonetheless be valuable, either as data from an observational cohort or as a comparison group with those who accepted randomization. Bothwell and Kesselheim (2017) advocate adaptive-design clinical trials, in which data are evaluated at interim points and then used to adapt study design, such as allocating more participants to better-performing arms of the study or dropping poorly performing arms altogether. This methodology has been "promoted as ethically advantageous over conventional RCTs because (it) reduce(s) the allocation of subjects to what appear to be inferior treatments" (Bothwell and Kesselheim 2017, 27). Herson notes that adaptive trials present unique challenges for monitoring committees: "The imbalance created by adaptive assignment may not permit adequate comparison of treatment groups for risk versus benefit" (Herson 2017, 169). Researchers might worry that such schemes would slow down recruitment of a randomized cohort or would slow the amassing of sufficient data to establish a clear signal about which arm is preferable. In light of these worries, there are significant ethical and statistical hurdles to some adaptive-design studies. Adaptive-design studies include the trade-off of exposing fewer participants to inferior treatment, but at the risk of needing to include greater numbers of participants in total, as participants are moved or dropped from poorly performing arms. In the case of the SIGHT trial, introducing an adaptative-design to bolster recruitment by reassuring potential participants that they would be moved to a better-performing arm mid-study, if evidence emerged that there was a better performing arm, would simultaneously create *greater barriers* to completion of the study by setting higher recruitment goals. Given that a major problem with the SIGHT trial was recruitment, and that the study was designed to allow participants the opportunity to eventually pursue treatment options outside of the ones in which they were initially randomized, it isn't clear that this revision would have helped. Despite these concerns, it remains worth asking, if so few participants would accept randomization, is this a sign that potential participants don't perceive the arms to be in equipoise, and thus there is something ethically questionable about the trial?

The semi-randomized, comprehensive cohort, or adaptive-design models are among many alternatives to the RCT that may be on the table. Alternatives to randomization can come with trade-offs. It is not incumbent on the ethicist in the DSMB to be familiar with all the alternatives to RCTs or the statistical details involved in drawing robust conclusions from each of these alternatives. But it is incumbent upon the ethicist to ask questions about the methodology, and alternative methodologies, especially when the methodology itself may be a barrier to the successful completion of a trial. DSMB members can pool their expertise to recommend alternative methodologies that answer clinical questions ethically, with statistically valid results. The DSMB has a responsibility to keep all participants safe and to ensure that their sacrifices in participating in research are worth the cost. The study that is stopped for lack of recruitment is just as undesirable as the study that is stopped because it fell out of equipoise.

Protecting Vulnerable Populations: DSMBs during COVID

Challenges to recruitment and the successful completion of trials may emerge not only when participants are reluctant to enroll but also when factors beyond the control of participants and researchers affect the viability of trials. Natural disasters, political upheaval, or armed conflict can undermine clinical trials. DSMBs may be overseeing multisite trials in which come recruitment sites may be faced with extreme challenges. One such challenge that affected clinical trials was COVID.

In early and mid-2020, during the "lockdown" phase of the COVID pandemic, one of the most fundamental ways in which research was affected concerned a revision in the balance of possible benefits and risks. Formerly "minimal risk" interventions, such as going to an in-person appointment to refill a medication, undergoing assessment for AEs, or undergoing routine tests to monitor study progress, became higher risk by virtue of being in-person. Many research participants were at additional risk of COVID owing to preexisting medical conditions. But even for participants who were otherwise healthy, or whose medical conditions did not put them at greater risk of COVID, in-person interactions were strongly discouraged. It was as if every participant became a member of a "vulnerable" population, overnight.[4]

Some research sites were closed to all but urgent clinical care. The responsibility of DSMBs is to protect research participants, but as shown by the SIGHT trial, in studies that aren't completed, benefits never outweigh risks. Thus, protecting the integrity of data collection was also foremost in the minds of DSMB members during COVID. On the NIH-sponsored studies whose DSMB's I served, researchers, representatives from the NIH, and members of DSMBs were in constant communication regarding trials already in progress. The studies could be grouped into three different types.[5]

The first were trials that were easily suspended. Resources at some sites—personal protective equipment and significant human resources—were at a premium. Many research sites suspended operations temporarily. Research participants were reluctant to attend visits even at sites that were operating at full capacity and, in many cases, were urged not to attend visits for their own protection. Some studies that had not yet met their enrollment goals had recruitment put on hold until a continuation of the trial was more tenable. DSMBs were rapidly consulted about trials that could be temporarily suspended.

The second type of trials were those that weren't suspended, but for which data collection could continue remotely or for which data collection could be pared down. Here, DSMBs had to work closely with sponsors to determine if continuing research remotely would put participants at greater risk or compromise data collection. Some types of data collection were easily moved to a remote setting, such as having a research assistant call a participant to fill out the fifty-item St. George's Respiratory Questionnaire over the phone. Pill counts could be similarly collected remotely or could wait until shelter-in-place orders were lifted. In some cases, AE collection could be tallied remotely. Other data collection, like a six-minute walk test used in the STRIVE study discussed in chapter 2, proved more challenging. Data collection might be imperfect, but the loss of benefit in quality of data had to be weighed against the harms to participants and burden on local investigators.

The third type of trials were ancillary studies added to trials of new drugs or therapies that might have treatment potential for COVID-19. Might therapies that were already being tested prove efficacious against the virus? DSMBs hastily reviewed informed consent addenda, and revised protocols, and mustered their expertise to assess the balance of benefit over risk in ancillary studies in which there were significant unknowns. It is notable that the quick responses required by DSMBs under the early weeks of the COVID-19 pandemic are anticipated in part by the FDA's own nonbinding guidance on DMCs, which says of some short-term trials with important safety concerns, "In order for the DMC to be informed and convened quickly in the event of unexpected results that raise concerns, special mechanisms would have to be developed to permit DMC evaluation and input" (U.S. Department of Health and Human Services 2006, 5). Might the FDA have anticipated that the quick mustering of monitoring committees might become necessary in routine trials suddenly beset by the extraordinary circumstances of the pandemic, and not only in short-term trials that might impose significant or unknown risk?

Four Lessons from COVID on How DSMBs Can Best Perform in Emergent Situations

Reflecting on the avalanche of work that resulted from the COVID pandemic, a few important lessons emerge. Although the lockdown stage of COVID is, we all hope, a thing of the past, the lessons learned from DSMB work during COVID can be adopted to other emergent situations in data safety monitoring.

The first lesson is to prioritize the protection of research subjects and primary endpoints, and triage secondary endpoints Some protocols' secondary endpoints read like a wish list, including myriad outcomes not necessarily connected to patients' priorities. Trialists would do DSMBs a service by being candid up front about the value of distinct secondary endpoints, letting the DSMB know which are formally statistically protected and which are part of a "wish-list" that can be jettisoned without compromising the possible benefits of the trial.[6] It is within the purview of the DSMB to ask for information about these secondary endpoints so that their statistical soundness and value to future patients can be reviewed. Rivera et al. endorse patient and public involvement with researchers in the "codevelopment of research," which would make research more ethical by both "democratizing the research agenda and/or helping to improve participant-facing documents and processes" (Rivera et al. 2022, 1915). These points mirror some of the concerns raised in chapter 2 in the discussion of patient advocates on DSMBs. Data collection that doesn't reflect participant priorities may be interesting to researchers but doesn't always outweigh the burden on participants. DSMBs occasionally found themselves recommending the unwelcome news that some research should not move forward as originally planned. Researchers should be ready to abandon some secondary

outcomes to focus on what really matters: protection of research participants in the quest to find treatments that will best serve participant cohorts
in the future. Even without a pandemic, some secondary endpoints are
luxury goods bought at the price of participants' time and exposure to risk.

**Second, rethink the balance of potential benefits and risks, especially in
light of the fact that data collection visits add costs to participants** Ethical research requires both that potential benefits exceed potential risks and
that risks are minimized as much as possible. As discussed in chapter 3, the
estimation of possible risks is an imperfect science, but the DSMB's members come to the table with expertise that allows them to make informed
judgments. The COVID lockdown required everyone to revisit risks in clinical trials and to make adjustments that maintained a positive balance of
possible benefits over risks. This is something DSMBs should have been
doing all long—overseeing collection of generalizable data that places the
smallest burden on participants.

Third, DSMBs should work in close communication with sponsors The
facts on the ground changed rapidly as a result of COVID. Sites that were
doing fine were suddenly inundated; sites that initially thought they
couldn't continue research later realized circumstances changed and they
were able to get back on track. DSMBs are used to being in close communication with sponsors, who relay information while allowing researchers to
maintain an unbiased distance. The pandemic furthered the importance of
this close communication. Heidi Ledford quoted Barbara Bierer, director of
the Multi-Regional Clinical Trials Center of Brigham and Women's Hospital
and Harvard: "Ethics committees are working overtime as researchers file
requests to alter their clinical-trial plans in ways that minimize how often
participants need to venture into the clinic" (Ledford 2020, 15). All DSMBs
should be set up to accommodate this rapid communication, even those
that don't typically require expedited communication of SAEs or similar
concerns. As seen in chapter 3, DSMBs may be called upon to recommend
revision to informed consent in the middle of studies; those recommendations may be tailored to different participants' circumstances. The need
to make recommendations about the revisions of informed consent, or to
consider recommendations about revisions of studies themselves, necessitates DSMBs remain in close communication with sponsors throughout
the research process. In 2005, when the DAMOCLES study group made its

recommendations, teleconference technology was neither as ubiquitous nor advanced as today. Thus, DAMOCLES recommended that data monitoring committees meet face-to-face rather than via teleconference. Today's DSMBs can meet remotely and come to quick decisions. Gordon, Sugarman, and Eass (1998) call for additional mechanisms that would allow for more seamless communication between DSMBs and IRBs. Going a step further, London and Kimmelman's (2019) endorsement of trial portfolios—trials that are interrelated by common objectives, such as testing similar articles that are evaluated together, and not in isolation—may argue for greater communication *among DSMBs*, many of which are simultaneously evaluating distinct trials with common objectives.

Finally, don't abandon your principles, even in the face of daunting challenges DSMBs are there to protect participants. In the rush to make changes during COVID, the protection of participants remained an essential job. Revised consent forms or procedures assembled by people who are under time pressure may leave out elements of informed consent. Revised informed consent documents should include all essential information; new procedures in ancillary studies should match those that are in consent forms, and vice versa. Even in the face of mounting external pressures, DSMBs are essential to protecting human subjects (Lou and Quin 2020). Despite the global need to find treatments and a vaccine as quickly as possible during the early stages of the lockdown, the responsibilities of researchers and DSMBs to trial participants remained intact (Maschke and Gusmano 2020). From the perspective of the DSMB members I worked with, and the sponsors to whom we communicated, if it took another few days for protections to be in place, it was worth it for the sake of participant safety.

The long-term lesson from the COIVD lockdown is that DSMBs were already doing an important job and already had the principles and skills to do that job in the midst of the unforeseen. DSMBs comprise hand-selected experts whose members have the unique clinical, statistical, and ethical background to oversee RCTs at their most dangerous period, when experimental treatments are actively given to brave volunteers and the effect of those treatments are being monitored. The ability to respond quickly, and the practical wisdom to apply expertise to a new emerging situation, is what data safety monitoring is all about.

After the initial lockdown phase, lingering effects of COVID continued to impact research. One of the long-term impacts of COIVD was its effect on the economy: initial loss of employment, which in the United States means loss of health care in many cases, working from home in some cases, supply-chain issues, and the so-called great resignation of people quitting jobs or exchanging their former jobs for those that afforded more compensation or flexibility. The direct impact of COVID on research was obvious: protective equipment used for research was abruptly repurposed for clinical care, and some data collection moved from in-person to remote methods, as discussed above. But the impact of the "great resignation" on participant recruitment and retention was also significant. Recruitment of participants, when done well, can be time-consuming, as it is based on forging relationships with potential participants. Without dedicated staff to help with recruitment, and consistency in recruitment, participant accrual can suffer. The turnover of research staff can have an impact on participant retention. In the SIGHT trial, one barrier to recruitment may have been a cultural disconnect, and possible perceived bias, between the potential participants and the researchers. Even if those gaps can be bridged, without consistency in the research space, participants can be discomforted. A lack of continuity among technicians who run tests can alienate participants. As research coordinators at local sites switch positions or spend more time working from home, retention of participants can suffer. Retention can be a "high touch" activity, requiring numerous personal contacts and continuous outreach to ensure participants feel connected to the research enterprise. Retention may be compromised if local sites are too busy to focus on research or lose staff whose job is to maintain close connections with participants. Attention to recruitment and retention is essential to ethical research; as stated above, the NIH 1998 guidelines recognize that monitoring "recruitment, accrual and retention" is within the DSMB's purview. DSMBs shouldn't be afraid to ask hard questions about budgeting that ensure these recruitment and retention activities aren't shortchanged.

Additional Steps Ethicists Can Take to Improve DSMB Oversight

In addition to the four lessons from COVID, there are additional steps that ethicists on DSMBs can take to promote participant safety throughout the research process.

Ensure the experiences of participants, especially marginalized participants, are adequately represented on the DSMB Some DSMB ethicists are asked to serve as both ethics expert and patient advocate. Dresser observes the experiences of research participants have been shortchanged in discussions of research ethics (Dresser 2017). The imaginative empathy cited in chapter 2 is an excellent first step, but it may take an ethicist only so far toward being an effective patient advocate. Dresser is correct when she notes (2017, xiii), "By considering actual subjects' perspectives, experts involved in the research enterprise can make more informed and ethical research decisions." Dresser's claims echo those of Adam Braddock, who cites the Agency for HealthCare Research and Quality's endorsement of "community-based participatory research (CBPR)." CBPR aims to integrate community members throughout the research process, "including selection of study topics, study design, participant recruitment, data collection, data analysis, and dissemination of research findings" (Braddock 2014, 81). Though not explicitly mentioned by Braddock, complementing the expertise on DSMBs with that of prior or current research participants would help contribute to these goals. Dresser's view (2017, xiv) is that "the failure to incorporate subjects' viewpoints into study planning and oversight decisions contributes to (the) current enrollment problems." Greater participant engagement in the development and oversight of research may result in projects that take into account the burdens and direct benefits of participation. This goal is shared by the Patient-Centered Outcomes Research Institute, which requires "research proposals it funds include patients and other stakeholders at every step of the research process," including development (Largent, Fernandez Lynch, and McCoy 2018, 7). Incorporating participants into the DSMB may have addressed enrollment problems that plagued the SIGHT trial. Dresser observes that although some of these steps to create greater community involvement will cost more in the short term, in the long run, there are significant benefits such as faster recruitment and higher participant retention (Dresser 2008, 234). Largent, Fernandez Lynch, and McCoy note that committees who would include patient participants should proceed with caution, as some of the "patient advocates" who are engaged in this role may be already well informed or networked with researchers, or inadequately trained to serve in these roles, or unrepresentative, as they are part of patient advocacy organizations that may not be representative. That is not to say that those patients' voices should not be heard. Largent, Fernandez Lynch, and McCoy offer several recommendations to better integrate patients into the decision-making process, including purposeful engagement of patient advocates who can be trained to take on this important role. When appropriate, ethicists should advocate for participant representation on DSMBs. In lieu of an actual patient partici- pant, ethicists should be mindful of taking seriously the dual role of both ethicist and patient advocate.

Work closely and respectfully with the other members of the DSMB to guide ethical decision-making Ethicists can prepare themselves to serve on a DSMB by doing background research on the diseases under study, diagnos- tic tests, and statistical methods. That preparation has its limits; the DSMB ethicists aren't there to be amateur clinicians or amateur statisticians. They are there to be professional bioethicists. Ethicists should use the expertise of the clinicians and statisticians to best understand what is happening in the research study or to best interpret results as the data emerges. Once those facts are understood, it is the job of the ethicist to find the ways to best pro- tect the interests of the participants, respect their autonomy, recommend conveying information via informed consent or a "re-consent" process, or interpret when risks and benefits are imbalanced. Ethicists can encourage other members of the DSMB to examine data in a new light or to examine how the equipoise of the study would be perceived from the point of view not only of researchers and the clinical community, but of participants and patients.

Ethicists should also be aware of themselves as ethicists, and the com- plexities that attend that role. These complexities may emerge in several ways. First, the technical terms that come with ethics training may be famil- iar to other ethicists but may be foreign to clinicians or statisticians on the DSMB. Ethicists should be respectful of other members of the committee by not obfuscating ethical concerns in needless jargon. Just as the complexities of a clinical trial can be conveyed in ordinary language in a consent form, the ethical complexities of a trial can be conveyed in ordinary language to members of the DSMB. Second, ethicists should be respectful of the way in which they engage other members of the DSMB so they don't come across as judgmental. Someone unfamiliar with high-level statistics might be called "innumerate." When someone is unfamiliar with high-level ethical nuance, do we call that person "unethical"? Surely not, yet ethicists should be wary of giving the impression that disagreement with their arguments doesn't render other members of the committee "unethical."[7] Ethicists carry a burden to not appear self-righteous, which leads to a third consideration. As pointed out in chapter 2, not all DSMBs have ethicists, and not all policy documents advocate including ethicists on DSMBs. Some policy recommendations, such as those offered by the DAMCOLES study group, were explicit in saying "no consensus was reached about ethicist or consumer or lay membership" on data monitoring committees (DAMOCLES 2005, 712). Reading between the lines, one can imagine that provocative back-and-forth may have emerged when the members of the DAMOCLES study group discussed the advisability of welcoming ethicists onto DSMBs. Ethicists on DSMBs are valuable contributors, albeit historically late additions to the DSMB guest list. Trial participants are best protected by a DSMB that has full appreciation of the history, policy, and theory that keeps them safe. As such, the continued presence by ethicists on DSMBs for studies characterized by uncertainty or risk is essential. Ethicists should be mindful of being constructive presences so they can perpetuate their role on DSMBs. Clinicians and statisticians are hand-selected for DSMBs because they bring unique backgrounds in the scientific and statistical methodologies utilized in the trials. Bioethicists can bring their unique background in the ethical complexities of clinical trials, as well as the ethical framework that guides DSMB work. That framework is the subject of the next chapter.

6 The Theoretical Foundations of DSMB Deliberations

Previous chapters considered the role of ethicists on DSMBs, what ethicists bring to the DSMB table, the weighing of risks and benefits by DSMBs, the unique role DSMBs have in revising informed consent documents during studies, questions surrounding equipoise, the role of DSMBs when trials involve vulnerable populations, and the unique challenges DSMBs faced when confronting the COVID pandemic. Every one of those topics merited its own ethical analysis. Underlying those issues remain assumptions about the overarching ethical framework that informs DSMB discussions.

This chapter presents a departure from the previous four chapters. Rather than recounting a trial that frames the debate, with an examination of specific ethical challenges that confront DSMBs, this chapter's focus is the theoretical underpinnings of clinical research ethics. Ethicists who serve on DSMBs should not only be familiar with the specifics of dealing with questions of informed consent or equipoise but also be equipped with a theoretical foundation that guides their overall thinking about the research enterprise. This is a more abstract endeavor than the previous chapters, but no less essential. For bioethicists acquainting themselves with DSMB work, some of the theories in research ethics will be familiar. For clinicians and statisticians who are learning about the role of ethicists on DSMBs, the discussion of ethical theories may be new, but their application to questions in research will be of interest. For non-ethicists, it is a valuable exercise to see where the ethicist at the DSMB table may be coming from.

The chapter argues for the claim that the ethic guiding clinical research is a consequentialist ethic, and thus, the ethic guiding DSMB deliberations is consequentialist. This is not a universally held view; the *Belmont Report*, Alex John London, and Emanuel, Wendler, and Grady have challenged this consequentialist approach. Consequentialist ethics argue that the consequences, ends, or results of an action determine the rightness or wrongness of that action. This ethic is one that argues that the rightness of wrongness of initiating, and of continuing, a trial is determined by the consequences that result from the trial. As such, the DSMB is integral to the project of ethical research—the DSMB scrutinizes the trial, not only before it commences but also *as it is taking place*, to ensure that the consequences of the trial continually justify the use of human participants. The DSMB, along with only a handful of individuals such as a medical monitor, have access to expedited SAE reports. Even then, the blinded medical monitor may not know the study arm of a participant who experienced an SAE or the wider context of an SAE report in light of additional study data. Although an unblinded statistician may have access to all the data, the DSMB is the only body with the responsibility of reviewing the entirety of the interim data in order to make a recommendation as to whether the study should continue. Consequences, like assessments of risk based on expedited SAE reports, or judgments about equipoise, are dynamic. Unexpected SAEs may be projected to be rare at a study's initiation, but that could change with time; a study that begins in equipoise may not always remain in equipoise. DSMBs are there to assess dynamic trials as they unfold, ensuring that studies are, and continue to be, ethical.

The Predominant View of Clinical Research Ethics

The National Commission, as stated in chapter 1, was instrumental in the creation of both the *policies* that guide human subjects research in the United States and the *ethical framework* that guides human subjects research. In 1979, the commission released "Ethical Principles and Guidelines for the Protection of Human Subjects of Research," colloquially known as the *Belmont Report*. The *Belmont Report* presents three ethical principles that guide the protection of human research participants: respect for the autonomy of persons, beneficence, and justice. The *Belmont Report*'s framework—a set of principles that jointly determine whether a particular course of action is morally right—is similar to the predominant bioethical theory in the United States today, set out in Tom Beauchamp and James F. Childress's *Principles of Biomedical Ethics* (2019). It is difficult to overestimate the impact of Beauchamp and Childress's contributions. To paraphrase another philosopher's observations about the use of ordinary language, the *Principles of Biomedical Ethics* isn't always the last word, but it is always the first word.[1]

Beauchamp and Childress lay out a theory of prima facie duties, in which four principles—the principle of respect for autonomy, beneficence, non-maleficence, and justice—guide our ethical thinking. They don't recognize a strict "principle-to-duty" correlation (Beauchamp and Childress 2019). Rather, actions are "in keeping" with principles. For example, respecting medical confidentiality is in keeping with the principle of respect for autonomy. The principles are prima facie principles, and not absolute, which is to say that no one of them consistently overrides any of the others (Beauchamp and Childress 2019). Instead, all relevant principles in any situation should be taken into account and weighed against each other in an attempt to reach a conclusion about the most ethical course of action. This weighing of the principles in an attempt to determine what is ethical is done by the process of *reflective equilibrium*. Informally, reflective equilibrium is an iterative process moving back and forth, from principles to specific cases, from specific cases to principles, until a point is reached at which no new information alters the conclusions as to what is right or correct. Beauchamp and Childress see reflective equilibrium both as a means of determining which principles are in keeping with the right action at any one time and as a method by which the four principles themselves are identified as the correct guide to bioethical decision-making. To take up the earlier example, respecting autonomy by maintaining confidentiality may not be the best course of action in some cases. For example, a duty of beneficence, such as a duty to protect persons in danger, may conflict with the promise of confidentiality in certain situations. Reflective equilibrium requires that a moral agent examine maintaining confidentiality as being in keeping with the principle of respect for autonomy; however, the agent also takes into account further information about protecting a person in danger, in keeping with the duty of beneficence. Information about a new set of obligations, in keeping with beneficence, might temper the agent's obligation that confidentiality be maintained. No one principle always takes precedence.

The *Belmont Report*, the document that guides ethical decision-making in research in the United States, is an example of a similar ethic of prima facie duties as that found in Beauchamp and Childress. The *Belmont Report* articulates three principles that guide ethical decision-making in research: ·

respect for persons, which incorporates both respecting the autonomy of agents who are autonomous, and protections for those who have diminished autonomy; beneficence, which incorporates obligations to not harm (nonmaleficence) and maximizing benefit; and justice, which incorporates concepts of equality, fairness, and dessert (National Commission 1979). Grady cites the contributions of LeRoy Walters in observing "since IRB review is a procedural mechanism for assuring that research complies with basic ethical principles and requirements, the primary criterion for judging the adequacy of any particular social control mechanism like an IRB is the extent to which it promotes the ethical principles" (Grady 2019, 36).

Given that Beauchamp and Childress's principlism theory is the predominant way of understanding bioethical questions in the United States today, and that the *Belmont Report* is the guiding policy document that lays out the ethical framework for human subjects research in the United States, on first glance it would appear uncontroversial to claim the moral theory that guides clinical research in the United States is an ethic of prima facie duties. A few notable holdouts disagree with this view. Benjamin Sachs rejects the ethical basis for common codes for decision-making in research ethics, such as the Nuremberg Code, Declaration of Helsinki, or *Belmont Report* (Sachs 2010). For Sachs, the *policies* that guide human research should not be confused with the *ethics* guiding human research. Instead, Sachs claims that many of the rules guiding research ethics are mere "starting points, subject to revision as the facts come in. Adopting this stance would constitute a long-overdue reorientation of our approach to rulemaking. It would mean embracing the idea of evidence-based rules in the arena of human subjects research" (Sachs 2010, 4). However, Sachs's view is a minority view. The authors of the *Belmont Report* contrast the report with codes of conduct such as Nuremberg, which presents a set of rules that "often are inadequate to cover complex situations; at times (they) come into conflict, and (they) are frequently difficult to interpret or apply" (National Commission 1979, 3). Rather than a set of rules that need to be followed, the *Belmont Report* articles three ethical principles that guide responsible research, part of the framework of prima facie duties.

This chapter argues that research on human beings is, in fact, not guided by an ethic of prima facie duties, but instead by a consequentialist ethic. Principles such as respect for autonomy, or justice, aren't to be discarded by DSMBs. But research itself is a *consequentialist* enterprise guided by *consequentialist* concerns. My view is that the ethicist on the DSMB is to look to consequentialist concerns when evaluating a study.

Establishing that human subjects research is a consequentialist endeavor requires a two-pronged argument. The first is a "negative" argument, an argument that shows that the ethic guiding human subjects research is *not* an ethic of prima facie duties. This is accomplished by looking carefully at one cornerstone of human subject research: informed consent. Obtaining informed consent from research subjects is said to be in keeping with the principle of respect for autonomy (Beauchamp and Childress 2019). According to the *Belmont Report*, "Respect for persons requires that subjects, to the degree that they are capable, be given the opportunity to choose what shall happen to them. This opportunity is provided when adequate standards for informed consent are satisfied" (National Commission 1979, 5). Informed consent is a means by which participant's authentic intention to be in research is protected by giving participants the relevant information they need to make a voluntary and informed choice based on their understanding of what is asked of them. However, when the need arises, this prima facie principle of autonomy, and the act of obtaining informed consent in keeping with autonomy, is jettisoned in clinical research for the sake of the principles of beneficence and nonmaleficence. In particular, the principle of autonomy is secondary to the promotion of beneficence and nonmaleficence *for groups*. In the case of promoting beneficence and nonmaleficence for groups in clinical research, those duties are held as more stringent prima facie principles than the principle of autonomy. However, the exchange is never made in the other direction: *It is never ethical in human research to forego beneficence and nonmaleficence for the sake of respect for autonomy*. The supposed "prima facie" nature of the principles doesn't hold up in the case of clinical research. Rather, prevention of risks and promotion of benefits for groups (both of which are part of the principle of beneficence), as well as non-affliction of harm (nonmaleficence), trump respect for autonomy. It cannot be the case that the principles are truly prima facie if the principles of beneficence and nonmaleficence may be viewed in some cases as more stringent than the principle of autonomy, but the principle of autonomy is *never* viewed as more stringent than beneficence and nonmaleficence.

At this point, a second step of the argument emerges. This step is a "positive" argument—an establishment of the ethic guides ethic clinical research. Rather than claim that clinical research is guided by competing prima facie principles, it is more accurate to say it is guided by an ethic that places the weighing of risks and benefits—and in particular, risks and benefits for groups—at the forefront. There is a name for an ethic that determines the moral normative status of actions based on the outcomes of an action, in particular the weighing of risks and benefit for groups: consequentialism.

A challenge emerges to the presumptive consequentialist framework of clinical research, in the form of the arguments posited by the anti-equipoise theorists. As discussed in chapter 4, maintaining equipoise is considered a necessary condition for ethical research by many. However, many bioethicists have forwarded arguments that challenge the primacy of equipoise. The arguments may be used to muster an objection to the claim that research ethics is fundamentally consequentialist. However, an examination of these arguments demonstrates that a consequentialist framework behind human research remains intact.

DSMBs are guided by this consequentialist framework. The argument demonstrates the centrality of ongoing monitoring of clinical trials, the primary work of DSMBs. Recognizing the centrality of DSMB work represents a call to reframe what it means to have ethical oversight of research. Overwhelmingly, the bioethical engagement in clinical trials has been trained on oversight *before projects commence*. The work of oversight of clinical research before the research begins is the responsibility of the researchers, the sponsors, the DSMB, and the IRB. As discussed in chapter 1, the primary responsibility of IRBs is to review protocols prior to the commencement of the research. Rather than casting most of our attention to the work that IRBs do—an ethical assessment *prior to the research even beginning*—bioethicists should reorient attention to an *ongoing ethical assessment throughout the research study*. Unlike the IRB, the DSMB has access to the entirety of the data during the course of a research study and thus is better positioned to make recommendations about the ethics of continuing studies as they progress. But before a conclusion can be drawn about where to fix our ethical attention in clinical research, an argument must first be made as to what its guiding ethic actually *is*.

The Voluntary Consent of the Human Subject Is Absolutely Essential . . . Except When It Isn't

An ethic of prima facie duties is executed in two steps. The first is to identify the competing prima facie duties in a given ethical dilemma. Expanding on the confidentiality example above, imagine a situation in which a psychiatric outpatient discloses to a counselor plans to kidnap an alleged nemesis. Should the counselor respect her patient's confidentiality, or does the counselor have a duty to warn the potential victim? The counselor had previously made a pledge of confidentiality to her patient. Respecting that pledge is owed to the patient, in keeping with the principle of respect for autonomy. The duty to prevent harm to the potential kidnap victim is in keeping with a duty of beneficence (recall that beneficence is about promoting benefit and preventing harm). This dilemma then is a conflict between Beauchamp and Childress's duties of respect for autonomy and beneficence. The second step is to then decide which of the competing prima facie duties is more "stringent" and act in keeping with the more stringent of those duties. In the above case, depending on the nature of the plans, whether the nemesis is an identifiable person, and if the only way to avoid significant harm is to violate confidentiality, a strong case could be made for violating confidentiality. Using this analysis, upholding the duty of beneficence to prevent harm to a third party is a more stringent obligation than upholding the duty to protect the patient's autonomy. However, if the harms were less significant (perhaps the claim about kidnapping was clearly an idle threat) or if there was a way to avoid harm without violating confidentiality, then acting in keeping with the principle of autonomy by upholding confidentiality may the more stringent duty. It is important to observe that there are some dilemmas about confidentiality in which autonomy takes precedence, and others in which beneficence takes precedence. An ethic of prima facie duties does not present a rank-ordering of duties. The duties are always weighed against each other; no one duty, or set of duties, is always more stringent than others.

If it were true that the ethic guiding clinical research were an ethic of prima facie duties, then it would *not* be the case that one principle, or set of principles, would always take precedence over another. And yet, that is precisely what happens.

Respect for autonomy is viewed as one of the prima facie principles guiding clinical research. Procuring informed consent is one action that is in keeping with this principle. Informed consent is a transformative tool in research ethics, as discussed in chapter 3. Heidi Li Feldman makes the important point that informed consent is valuable because it affirms the "separateness of persons [which] signals the differences between different people's ends and the distinctiveness of what goes into each person's flourishing" (Feldman 2014, 304). Not all persons have the same goals, plans, and values. It may be that researchers have different objectives from their research participants. The therapeutic misconception, therapeutic mis-estimation, and unrealistic optimism cited in chapter 5 are three of many ways in which research participants may evidence different objectives in their participation in research—such as expectation of direct therapeutic benefit—than researchers. Informed consent is that piece of the puzzle that bridges the gap between the researchers' understanding of their goals and values in performing research and the participants' understanding of their role in research.

However, there are significant instances in which informed consent is waived, or done away with altogether, because the principles of beneficence and nonmaleficence are viewed as more stringent. To present the strongest argument possible, I will leave aside examples of research in which the stakes are so low that informed consent can be waived, per the Common Rule. For example, research on public behavior, such as observing whether people altruistically return shopping carts to designated areas, does not require informed consent from participants. Similarly, deception research that is minimal risk and could not be practicably carried out without a waiver of informed consent is also permissible. An example of such deception research includes a psychological study evaluating levels of frustration of participants told they are playing a computer game in remote collaboration with another person but are in fact playing with a computer programmed to undermine their efforts. If the participants were told that they were playing a rigged game, their levels of frustration could not be adequately measured; thus, this study could not be accomplished without a waiver of informed consent; however, the minimal risk of harm may be justified. Research that promises merely "de minimis risk," as put forward by Rosamond Rhodes, may similarly afford cases in which "informed consent should not be considered an absolute requirement for the ethical conduct of human subjects research" (Rhodes 2014, 41). Minimal risk or "de minimis risk" research doesn't make the most persuasive case.

Gelinas, Wertheimer, and Miller (2016) present two grounds upon which research without consent may be permissible. They first include (2016, 35) "socially valuable research [which] is justified without the consent of the participants if the research stands to infringe no right of the participants and it is impracticable to obtain consent." The second includes "research that does infringe participants rights [which] can be justified if the gravity of the rights infringement is minor and outweighed by the expected social value of the research and it is impracticable to obtain consent" (2016, 36). Gelinas, Wertheimer, and Miller present four examples of research that meet these two requirements; only the last of these four examples is an RCT. Their argument is that consent is employed in situations in which an agent waives a "right of control"—consent is needed when one agent is at risk of harming another agent by violating their sovereignty or right of control over themselves. Thus, if no right is violated, then no consent is morally required. Additionally, rights are not absolute—they can and should be weighed against other considerations. If a right of sovereignty or control is violated by a failure to obtain consent, but a greater good is served, that state of affairs may be morally permissible. Although not all of Gelinas, Wertheimer, and Miller's examples engage the types of studies that may be overseen by DSMBs, their arguments and conclusions about clinical research are consistent with the argument being made here—namely, that clinical research is guided by an ethic that places risks and benefits at the forefront, allowing autonomy to be compromised if necessary. They maintain that if their conclusions hold, "[the] idea that informed consent constitutes a foundational norm of human research requires substantial qualification" (Gelinas, Wertheimer, and Miller 2016, 36).

Finally, to further the argument, I also leave aside controversial cases, such as the one set out by Truog et al. (1999) or Faden et al. (2013), who argue that informed consent to research can be waived in the special circumstance in which a trial compares two medically indicated treatments, or comparative effectiveness trials such as "checklist" protocols.

The cases discussed below are cases of research that *exceed minimal risk* or are not merely comparing a known treatment to another known treatment. The stakes are higher, and yet autonomy isn't always adequately protected. All are examples of "the numerous exceptions under which research may be undertaken without the consent of its subjects" (Capron 2014, 145). Additionally, these are not cases in which informed consent is found to be inadequate, imperfect, or not ideal. Informed consent rarely lives up to its ideal. These are not cases of the perfect being the enemy of the good. Rather, these arguably are cases of ethical research conduct in the *absence of informed consent,* imperfect though it may be. If the risks are properly man-aged, and the benefits are considered high enough, then informed consent is not always required.

Research on people who cannot give informed consent   Research is done on children, persons with cognitive impairments that may affect decision-making, and persons who were previously competent to offer informed consent, but no longer are, such as persons with dementia. This is merely a partial list of persons who cannot give informed consent and yet are used in clinical research. The justification for this research usually incorporates the principles of justice, beneficence, and autonomy. First, it is an injustice for research not to take place on childhood leukemia, adult schizophrenia, or Alzheimer's disease because without research, beneficial new therapies for these conditions would never be discovered. This justification cites both the principles of justice and beneficence to support research on people who cannot autonomously consent. However, some nod to autonomy is also made: in many of these cases, researchers rely on assent from the partici-pants. Assent requires affirmative agreement without requiring the robust expectations of voluntariness, competency, and understanding that charac-terizes informed consent. Informed consent in these instances is obtained from surrogate decision-makers—parents, adult children, or other LARs. It can be argued that surrogate decision-making is, in fact, informed consent by virtue of the fact that these research participants cannot consent on their own. But there is certainly a difference between relying on the consent of a surrogate and relying on the actual consent of the research participant. Surrogate consent is, at best, second to obtaining actual consent from the research participant. Consider, for example, a case in which a participant denies assent but the surrogate offers consent. In cases in which a potential participant's lack of assent conflicts with a surrogate's consent to research participation, we don't automatically allow the surrogate's informed con-sent to override the lack of assent. Consent from surrogates doesn't always carry the day—it is not the same as receiving the participant's consent and should not be mistaken for such. Thus, in these cases, the principles of justice and beneficence are upheld, as is autonomy, but to a lesser degree.

Perhaps this case isn't entirely persuasive because the principle of auton-omy is represented by the surrogate's determination, especially in cases of a substituted judgment on behalf of a less-than-autonomous participant—hence the need for additional, more persuasive examples.

Research on persons in the military   Some research on people in the military does not require the protection of informed consent (Parasidis 2014). Research in the military must first be evaluated for risks and benefits so beneficence and nonmaleficence are upheld, but in lieu of informed consent, there is no provision for protecting autonomy. According to Bonham and Moreno, "The command and control framework of military operations means that solider-participants can be ordered to participate in activities like research or find themselves the recipients of an experimental product administered without their knowledge when their supervisors determine that the action is necessary to protect the safety of the force or to accomplish military goals" (2008, 469). For example, some Department of Defense protocols "allow for an informed consent waiver if instances where the President determines that national security interests justify force-wide nonconsensual use for off-label or investigational products" (Parasidis 2014, 68). Bonham and Moreno cite the example of experimental vaccines against biological and chemical weapons that were administered during the Gulf War without consent from soldiers, but with an emergency waiver of informed consent issued by the FDA: "After lengthy internal and inter-agency discussions, the FDA agreed and in December 1990 issued new, interim regulation to permit the military to administer investigational drugs and biologics to military personnel without obtaining informed consent" (Bohman and Moreno 2008, 471). It might be argued that people serving in the military cannot be entirely autonomous, which is why informed consent is unnecessary. The institutional nature of the military precludes true informed consent, so why even engage in the fiction of obtaining informed consent? This argument might be persuasive, except that there are examples of research in settings whose institutional structures significantly undermine autonomy, which nonetheless *do* require informed consent. The Common Rule presents detailed requirements for performing research on people in prison. Additional protections exist for research participants in prisons *beyond those for persons who are not imprisoned*, in part because prisoners' autonomy is believed to be compromised.[2] Presumably, the autonomy of *volunteers* in the military is at least as great as those who are *involuntarily* imprisoned. Thus, the argument that informed consent in the military is a fiction because of the institutional nature of the military is not persuasive—people in the military have at least as much autonomy as those in prison, and prisoners do have the right to informed consent prior to serving in clinical research.

Another argument against the need for informed consent from those serving in the military is that they have already given informed consent to participate in research. By autonomously signing up to serve in the military, anyone who serves already agrees to any activity that the military asks, including serving as a research subject. This may be a more persuasive argument, but only slightly. The argument relies on the claim that if an agent autonomously agreed to an action, that agent autonomously agrees to any additional actions the agreed-upon action entails, even if the agent was not told what those additional actions were at the time of initial agreement. This claim is questionable, though, because it relies on the inconsistency of saying that an agent *autonomously* agreed to something without knowing the consequences (viz: not having sufficient knowledge to be autonomous) of that to which they were agreeing. Furthermore, this is inconsistent with what informed consent to clinical research looks like in practice, as illustrated by chapter 3's discussion of a DSMB's deliberations in recommending revision of informed consent mid-study. If a research protocol changes in ways that alter the risks to participants, or if new information is made available that would further inform a subject's voluntary choice to enroll in a study, participants are often offered the new information and are asked to again offer informed consent to participation. In most cases, as facts about the risks of an intervention change, and those risks have an impact on participants, the participants in the research study should be told about that changing risk profile. The idea of a "blanket" consent, in which mere agreement to be in an institution (such as the military) is ethically sufficient to count as autonomous consent to clinical research, doesn't stand up. It cannot be said that clinical research on members of the military upholds autonomy, even though the principles of beneficence and nonmaleficence are upheld through requirements that the research is scrutinized for medical value and risk minimization.

In light of the limits of autonomy among members of the military, Parasidis argues for more extensive protections for military members in research. These additional protections consist of classifying members of the military as "vulnerable subjects" in the same vein as prisoners, per the Common Rule; including IRB representatives who have military experience to act as participant advocates for research on military members; strengthening informed consent protections; and including "consent monitors" to assess decision-making and voluntariness of potential participants (Parasidis

2014, 73–75). Until those changes are put into effect, however, research in military settings remains an example in which the principle of respect for autonomy is less stringent than beneficence and nonmaleficence.

Research during terrorism or other public health emergencies   Effective June 2011, it is legal to use some experimental diagnostic measures on people without their consent during some forms of attack or other public health emergencies (including pandemics). According to the Code of Federal Regulations 21 CFR 50.23(e),

> Obtaining informed consent for investigational in vitro diagnostic devices used to identify chemical, biological, radiological, or nuclear agents will be deemed feasible *unless* [italics mine], before use of the test article, both the investigator (e.g., clinical laboratory director or other responsible individual) and a physician who is not otherwise participating in the clinical investigation make the determinations and later certify in writing all of the following:
>
> (i) The human subject is confronted by a life-threatening situation necessitating the use of the investigational in vitro diagnostic device to identify a chemical, biological, radiological, or nuclear agent that would suggest a terrorism event or other public health emergency.

Additional items (ii), (iii), and (iv) include that there is no way for the patient to know an experimental intervention was the only one available, that there isn't sufficient time to obtain consent without the patient's life being in danger, that there isn't sufficient time to obtain consent from a LAR, and that there is no non-experimental method of diagnosis available at the time. During a public health emergency, informed consent for research on diagnostic tests can be waived, even for persons who are competent to give consent. The reasoning behind this waiver is that during a public health emergency it is imperative to develop accurate diagnoses of as many people as possible; as such, both testing experimental diagnostic procedures and, ideally, receiving accurate diagnoses from those still-experimental procedures is necessary. This is a clear instance in which the duty to protect autonomy, in the form of informed consent from research participants, is perceived as secondary to promoting the greatest good for the populace.

A possible response to the use of this example is that the use of biological material for an in vitro medical test, especially during a terrorist attack or other health emergency, is surely outweighed by the benefits; as such, a usurpation of autonomy here is entirely appropriate. But notice this is an argument that precisely proves the point: considerations of harm and benefit should be paramount, rather than protection of autonomy. Even in cases in which a patient is able to give informed consent to experimental diagnostic procedures, considerations of risk and benefit to the population are more fundamental than those of autonomy. A second response is that such interventions are minimal risk and, as such, undermine the argument. The harms from a blood draw or other noninvasive tests are so small as to not effectively prove the point about autonomy being outweighed by considerations of beneficence and nonmaleficence. However, the claim that these articles may convey only the minimal risks of routine blood draws or similar collection procedures fails to take into consideration the harms of false positive or false negative test results. A lot is at stake when diagnosing a patient during a terrorist attack or public health emergency. But so too, a great deal is at stake in *misdiagnosing* someone under those circumstances. The FDA, in codifying 21 CFR 50.23, asserted that the balance of risks and harms is more significant than the autonomy rights of the patient to decide for themselves whether to accept the risks of the false negative or false positive from a still-experimental test. As such, this may well be another example of a case of clinical research in which considerations of beneficence and nonmaleficence outweigh those of autonomy.

Research in emergent circumstances Federal regulations allow for a waiver of informed consent for some types of research in emergent situations (Grady 2015). Informed consent may be waived when it is impossible to obtain consent from participants, no surrogate is on hand to offer consent, and there is a narrow therapeutic window in which to administer the experimental therapy. Additional requirements include that the experimental therapy is only for the condition for which the participant was admitted to the hospital, there is no accepted standard of care for the condition, and the experimental therapy is reasonably expected to be of direct benefit to the participant. In a review of twenty years of studies that employed either an exemption from informed consent or a waiver of informed consent, Klein, Moore, and Biros (2018) found that forty-five such studies had been conducted—the greatest number for cardiac arrest (ten studies), hemorrhagic shock (six studies), and traumatic brain injury (five studies)—with a finding that 63,974 patients had been enrolled in such studies (Klein, Moore, and Biros 2018, 1172). Regulations require that researchers attempt to obtain informed consent after the fact and that the community in which the research is being done is consulted prior to the research (Klitzman 2015, 121). However, these "post-hoc" attempts at "informed consent," including community-wide consultations, are poor substitutes for protecting participant autonomy via true informed consent. Furthermore, according to Klein, Moore, and Biros's findings, whether these provisions are followed is inconsistently reported in the literature. So why even sanction this type of research, in which neither informed consent from the research participant nor surrogate consent from an authorized representative is required? It is because there are some therapies for emergent conditions that require a narrow therapeutic window in which they are administered and can only be tested during that brief period of time. If researchers had to rely on the accrual of research participants only in cases in which people with emergent conditions presented with surrogates on hand, the expectation is that the development of some therapies for those conditions—some interventions for cardiac arrest, hemorrhagic shock, or traumatic brain injury, as listed above—would be prohibitively delayed. Emergent research is thus another instance in which considerations about risks and benefits outweigh the need for informed consent prior to enrollment in a clinical trial.

In summary, there are several examples in which the principles of beneficence and nonmaleficence are elevated over the principle of autonomy, protected via informed consent, in clinical research. Capron refers to the moral justification of these cases as "the lure of utility" (2014, 149), observing that "we keep venerating informed consent, all the while looking for ways to conduct more and more research without it" (151). Feldman laments that utilitarianism, along with libertarianism, is a threat to the separateness of persons (Feldman 2014). Utilitarianism focuses too much on aggregate goals to the exclusion of the interest of individuals, whereas libertarianism focuses on each individual's goals to the exclusion of other individual's interests. Whether this is, in fact, a lamentable position will be considered later. For now, the lesson is that practices such as informed consent, in keeping with the principle of autonomy, can be overridden for the sake of beneficence and nonmaleficence.

However, *there are no corresponding asymmetries*: there are no cases in which research is permitted to go forward, even with informed consent, absent the expectation of a positive balance of possible benefits over potential risks. Imagine the researchers who professed, "We knew nothing of scientific or therapeutic value could possibly come from this poorly designed and ill-conceived experiment, but participants gave informed consent, so it was permissible to perform the study." Such a study would not be viewed as ethical.

Objectors to the claim that there are no corresponding asymmetries may point to cases of "challenge studies," in which, for example, a participant is intentionally infected with a disease so that possible treatments for the disease can be studied. Debates about the ethical permissibility of challenge studies emerged during the pandemic, as the need to test and approve vaccines quickly became a global concern (Fernandez Lynch et al. 2021; Jamrozik and Selgelid 2020). Might challenge studies be a counterexample to the claim that the balance of benefits and risks is paramount in clinical research, superseding concerns about autonomy? The autonomous challenge study participant agrees to place themselves at risk of harm by being exposed to a disease to test if a vaccine or treatment is successful. However, even in this case, the point of the challenge study is that the *overall* expectation of benefit—a vaccine that could be available to millions and millions of people—is greater than the expectation of harm to the research participants. The poorly designed, methodologically flawed challenge study wouldn't be ethical, no matter how informed the consent from its voluntary human participants may be. Even when autonomy is protected via informed consent, that is not sufficient to overcome a state of affairs in which the benefits of research are outweighed by the potential harms.

Another objection may be raised based on the work of Robert M. Veatch (2009). Veatch, among the "anti-equipoise" theorists discussed below, argues that the assessment of the individual physician or member of the clinical or scientific community is not what determines the moral permissibility of enrolling a participant into a randomized study. The indifference, ambivalence, or preference among competing arms on the part of experts isn't relevant, owing both to the fact that absolute indifference is rare and the fact that clinicians and researchers may have idiosyncratic preferences among treatment arms (Veatch 2009). Veatch instead contends that justifications for randomization must be based on the indifference of potential participants. Take, for example, the three-arm SIGHT trial, in which therapies researchers held to be in equipoise before the trial began—drug therapy, one type of surgery, a second type of surgery—were therapies among which patients may have had decided preferences. Time devoted to treatment,

AEs, and recovery time are all borne by participants, and each participant may have individual assessments of the potential benefits and harms that obtain. As such, it is the *participant's judgment alone* that justifies enrollment into a randomized trial. Veatch concludes, "A clinician is morally justified in entering a patient into a randomized clinical trial if, and only if, that individual patient after being adequately informed is approximately indifferent between the two treatment options or is otherwise willing to take the risk of receiving what to him or her is the less attractive option" (2009, 211). It should be the participant's choice to engage in research; a participant's view of the potential benefits and harms of the trial are fundamental to determining whether the study is ethical. This is the lesson of E7, discussed in chapter 4, an admirable and perhaps uncontroversial claim. A second claim, though, is striking: Veatch proposes that a randomized study is morally justified *if and only if* a patient is indifferent after being informed about the nature of the study. The claim is that patient indifference is both necessary and *sufficient* for randomization into a study. Is Veatch arguing that patient preference alone, on the basis of informed consent, is both necessary and sufficient for ethical research, thereby arguing against my claim that principles of autonomy are never outweighed by considerations of beneficence or nonmaleficence? I don't believe that this is what Veatch meant; this reading is both too broad and uncharitable. Veatch is not arguing that patient indifference, as articulated after being informed, is *sufficient* for all research to be ethical. Rather, the participant's agreement is sufficient and necessary for randomization.

Veatch recounts the lessons of monitoring an open-label study of two treatments for childhood leukemia. One of the potential participants was devastated to learn she had been randomized to her nonpreferred treatment arm. Veatch reflected on the lessons of this experience—that clinician and researcher indifference among study arms could not have been determinative of ethical randomization. Instead, "if patients, after being informed, have a subjective preference for the standard treatment, they should get it" (Veatch 2009, 214). Veatch argues that placing participants in a given arm of a study, without their consent to that specific arm, is morally unacceptable. However, although he finds *randomization* without consent unacceptable, Veatch is not going so far as to say that autonomous choice outweighs considerations of potential benefit or harm in research. His claim about randomization should not be taken as a claim that autonomous decision-making is sufficient for ethical research, in the absence of expected direct or aspirational benefits. Thus, although Veatch argues for centrality of participant preferences in randomization, it isn't clear that those considerations extend to those cases of clinical research conducted without informed consent, discussed above.

There are exceptions in which respect for autonomy, as executed via informed consent, is outweighed by the potential benefits of the trial. When it comes to clinical research, upholding the principles of beneficence and nonmaleficence is necessary, and in some cases sufficient, for a study to move forward. Promoting the principle of respect for autonomy is not always necessary, and it is *never sufficient*, for research to move forward.

This asymmetry shows that the ethic of human research is *not* an ethic of prima facie duties. If it were truly an ethic of prima facie duties, there would be instances in which the principles of beneficence and nonmaleficence would be more stringent than the principle of autonomy, *and* vice versa. However, there are no cases in which the principle of respect for autonomy can overcome a situation in which the harms of research are expected to exceed the benefits. The principles of beneficence and nonmaleficence—to promote good in clinical research and to prevent harm, both to current research participants and to future cohorts of those participants who will gain from the generalizable knowledge that results—take precedence every time.

A position on the subordination of informed consent to considerations of benefit and risk is put forward by David Wendler (2011). His view is that "investigators should be permitted to enroll participants when they have sufficient evidence that the participants have provided valid informed consent" (Wendler 2011, 1587). Wendler's position is that consent from participants is a necessary condition for the permissibility of clinical trials. What counts as "valid informed consent"? For Wendler, the answer depends on the risks and benefits that the participants are expected to experience by virtue of their trial participation. In studies with low risks, the threshold for determining competence, understanding, and voluntariness is lower. In studies with high risks, either those that offer the potential for direct benefit or offer little or no potential direct benefit, formal assessments of understanding or voluntariness may be required. The lower the risks, the lower the threshold for determining if autonomy is protected; the higher the risks, the higher the threshold for determining if autonomy is protected. In other words, the scope of autonomy protections afforded by informed consent may be determined by first establishing the risks and benefits of study participation. According to Wendler, the principle of respect for persons, upheld by the practice of informed consent, while necessary to the practice of responsible research, is nonetheless subordinate to—subordinate to the point of *being determined by*—principles of beneficence and nonmaleficence.

The ethic of human research is an ethic in which the obligations to promote good and prevent harm are paramount. It is an ethic whose foremost focus is on the outcomes of the research. Ethical theories in which the outcomes of certain actions determine their moral normative status are consequentialist theories. The ethic of clinical research appears to be a consequentialist ethic, and not the ethic of prima facie duties expounded by the *Belmont Report*, or Beauchamp and Childress.

Clinical Research and a Consequentialist Ethic

Should we bite the bullet and accept that the ethic of human research is a consequentialist ethic? The claim that human research is guided by a consequentialist ethic is not new. Franklin G. Miller and Howard Brody (2003) support the view that clinical research is fundamentally utilitarian, a version of consequentialism: "Clinical research is dedicated primarily to promoting the medical good of future patients by means of scientific knowledge derived from experimentation with current research participants—a frankly utilitarian purpose" (Miller and Brody 2003, 21). Elsewhere, Miller and Brody claim that "a basic feature of clinical research ethics is utilitarian or consequentialist" (Miller and Brody 2007,162). Miller and Brody's argument is based on their dismissal of the "similarity position"—that the ethics of clinical care and the ethics of clinical research are similar. The similarity position is mistaken, in their view, because the goals of clinical care and clinical research are distinct. This argument is one that rejects the ethics of "personal care"—the second type of argument presented in chapter 4 for the centrality of equipoise. Such arguments hold that the duties of personal care that physicians owe their patients are akin to the duties researchers owe their participants. For this reason, Miller and Brody reject equipoise as a necessary condition for ethical research; the ethical requirement of equipoise is predicated on the erroneous conflation of the ethics guiding clinical care and the ethics guiding clinical research. It appears that biting the consequentialist bullet requires a significant trade-off—accepting that research is a consequentialist enterprise means abandoning equipoise. In the following section, this anti-equipoise argument will be taken up.

A comparable claim to Miller and Brody's, that clinical research is a consequentialist enterprise, is put forward by Paul Litton and Franklin G. Miller (2005). They examine whether the ethic that guides clinical medicine—one grounded in Beauchamp and Childress's principles, and, in particular, the principle of beneficence toward individuals, for example—is the same ethic that guides clinical research. They present multiple arguments to conclude that the ethic guiding clinical research is *not* the same as that guiding clinical medical practice. Their first argument is based on Thomas Scanlon's contractualist position that we ought to act from "principles for the general regulation of behavior that others, similarly motivated, could not reasonably reject" (Scanlon 1998, 4). This principle, grounded in the mutual respect that ought to be shared among all persons, would yield certain conclusions on the part of current and potential research participants. Since research is about the creation of generalizable knowledge, and since so many current and potential research participants stand to benefit from that knowledge, "it follows that the distinctive goal of research *is* normatively significant: there are good reasons to design research protocols for the purpose of producing socially important, generalizable medical knowledge" (Litton and Miller 2005, 568, emphasis theirs). Current and potential research participants would agree to the normative emphasis of research being the promotion of benefits and reduction of harm for groups, and not merely individuals—this is a principle that others, similarly motivated, could not reasonably reject.

Litton and Miller observe that although research participants might be on board with these claims, perhaps the researchers themselves would balk, thinking the ethical orientation of research ethics, when distinct from the ethical orientation of clinical medicine, is not sufficiently focused on the value of research participants as persons. Might the orientation of research ethics be *too* focused on the promotion of benefit and reduction of harm for groups, and not adequately focused on respect for persons, to satisfy the responsible physician-investigator? Litton and Miller at this juncture make use of the seven requirements for ethical research put forward by Emanuel, Wendler, and Grady (2000), each of which "expresses a respectful attitude towards the worth of each patient-subject" (Litton and Miller 2005, 569).

These seven requirements include 1) risks to subjects must be reasonable, 2) the research has social value, 3) the research is scientifically valid, 4) subjects give free and informed consent, 5) subject selection is fair, 6) the research undergoes independent review, and 7) the research is consistent with "respect for persons." Litton and Miller hold that when these seven requirements are met, investigators are treating participants with respect. To assume a more therapeutic stance—to go beyond these seven requirements *and* expect that participants be given their best treatment option even within a clinical trial—paternalistically overstates the vulnerability of research participants. The upshot is that the requirement of equipoise, in which no participant is disadvantaged by their participation in any arm of a study, is not required for clinical research to be ethical. The ethics of personal care is too paternalistic to be a reasonable guide to ethical clinical research.

A second argument offered by Litton and Miller is that it is unduly paternalistic for research participants to be forbidden from relinquishing their access to "the best care" in favor of serving in research. Given the seven requirements above, including informed consent and fair subject selection, shouldn't people have the right to participate in trials, even if participation deprives them of optimal care? The claim here is that depriving potential participants of this right is predicated on a misguided "therapeutic orientation" in clinical trials. Litton and Miller here may be describing the case of "bad choice" studies described by Menikoff and Richards (2006, 68). This "therapeutic orientation ignores that persons have reason to want the ways in which they are treated depend on the choices they make, especially when placed in a sufficiently good position to make an informed decision" (Litton and Miller 2005, 571). Perhaps participants have other values—the desire to give back to others, altruism, or gratitude—that might be more significant than personal medical benefit. The therapeutic orientation embraces a paternalism that Litton and Miller find objectionable. Again, notice that the upshot of this type of argument is a rejection of equipoise as a necessary condition for the ethical clinical trial, as it shows that randomization that results in a participant in a less-optimal arm of a study is ethically permissible.

Litton and Miller do not explicitly claim that the ethic behind clinical research is a consequentialist one. Rather, they merely claim that the ethic that guides clinical research is distinct from the personal care model used in clinical practice. They do make clear that the ethic of clinical care is based on promotion of benefit and reduction of harm for individuals, whereas the ethic of clinical research is about the promotion of benefit and reduction of harm *for groups*. Although they don't call this "consequentialism" directly, one is hard-pressed to know what else to call it. It is notable that Litton and Miller cite Scanlon's *contractualist* theory to bolster what appears to be the claim that research is a primarily *consequentialist* enterprise. Litton and Miller take pains to show that Scanlon's theory "is meant to expose the deeper normative assumptions behind the forthcoming arguments"—that is, his contractualist theory, based on the respect owed all persons, may point the way to a consequentialist foundation for research ethics.

Alex John London is another bioethicist who reflects on whether clinical research is an inherently utilitarian enterprise. London disagrees, dismissing the utilitarian claim as one of the "Two Dogmas of Research Ethics" (London 2007b). London examines the explicit utilitarian views of Miller and Brody as well as the more implicit utilitarian assumptions woven through the history of research ethics. Given these utilitarian assumptions, London maintains that one of the "dogmas" of clinical research is that it is guided by utilitarianism. The second dogma is that any additional duties imposed upon researchers are mere "side constraints" to the utilitarian agenda, side constraints that emerge from role-related obligations.

According to London, clinical research emerged from a medical tradition with roots in Hippocratic thinking, one that promotes explicit duties to patients. The role-related duties of researchers to participants have a history in the role-related duties of health-care providers to patients. Take, for example, Emanuel, Wendler, and Grady's above-cited seven requirements of ethical research. London observes that the first three of these requirements are not *side-constraints* on a utilitarian ethic—they are an *articulation* of a utilitarian ethic. These three requirements must be fulfilled for clinical research to maximize utility for all parties concerned. The claim that research ethics is not utilitarian is off to a rocky start. Additionally, the remaining four "side constraints" are not inconsistent with a utilitarian ethic and, in fact, can be supported by a rule utilitarian ethic. Policies requiring informed consent to most research or fair subject selection—most often associated with the prima facie principles of respect for autonomy and justice, respectively—can be justified by the fact that utility is maximized when such policies are put into place, so as to bolster the reputation of the research enterprise. Participants who voluntarily consent to serve in research are more likely to adhere to what may be an onerous research protocol, and thus, utility is maximized when consent is obtained. Imagine what may have happened in the SIGHT protocol, discussed in chapter 5, if participants were able to voluntarily choose and consent to an arm of the study rather than being randomized.

London similarly believes that the therapeutic misconception can be understood as a type of "patient-centered consequentialism"—a mistaken belief that even in the research context, researchers have a duty to "advance the interests of the individual patient" (London 2007b, 104). There are many ways to demonstrate that Emanuel, Wendler, and Grady's four last requirements are justified using consequentialist reasoning. The "second dogma of research ethics"—that the side constraints placed on an explicitly utilitarian ethic are justified by *nonutilitarian claims*—does not hold up. These side constraints are either themselves explicitly consequentialist or are at the very least, compatible with a consequentialist ethic.

What, then, of the first dogma of research ethics—the claim that the ethic that guides clinical research, even absent the "side-constraints," is a utilitarian ethic? London's view is that clinical research actually *rejects* two essential aspects of utilitarianism, and thus, clinical research is not guided by utilitarianism. The first utilitarian assumption is that goodness consists of the utility experienced by persons, understood as the welfare of individuals ("welfarism"). The second is that the goodness of states of affairs is based on the sum total of utility that results from said states of affairs ("sum-ranking"). Welfarism and sum-ranking may result in maximizing utility for the aggregate of persons, but welfarism and sum-ranking alone fail to take into account equality among persons; similarly, they do not allow for the possibility that some equalities should never be breached.

London instead endorses an "Integrative Approach" (IA) based on both John Rawls's view that there exist a set of basic interests that should not be compromised, coupled with a capacities approach that sets parameters as to what those basic interests are (London 2007a and 2007b). London believes clinical research is best understood within IA's framework. IA both better justifies the goals of clinical research and offers a justification for the "side constraints" discussed above. Clinical research is thus not justified on the basis of utilitarian claims—what will benefit the group to the greatest degree. Neither the Rawlsian view nor the capacities approach is about ensuring that primary social goods or human capacities are *maximized*. Rather, there are basic minimums that everyone ought to be accorded. Clinical research "is viewed as one element within a larger social division of labor that must be justifiable to the individual community members whose interests that division of labor is supposed to safeguard and advance" (London 2007b, 110).

IA is a coherent and attractive position insofar as it recognizes that persons deserve a basic minimum of decent treatment while at the same time accounting for fair treatment and just distribution of benefits and burdens. It isn't clear, however, that London has established that clinical research is appropriately guided by the IA ethic. We must examine clinical research itself—its practices and goals—to establish which ethic best informs its practices. Not every human activity will have the same practices and goals; some activities seem better matched to a Rawlsian and capacities-based view than others. *Primary education*, for example, would seem to be an excellent candidate for an IA ethic. Human flourishing is best achieved when people have a certain level of autonomy and the ability to appreciate certain experiences to their fullest. Given that human flourishing is associated with education, there should be a basic minimum of education that every child receives. *Health care* may also be a strong candidate for IA; without a basic minimum of health care, human capacities go unfulfilled. Is *clinical research* a good candidate for London's approach? One important distinction between clinical research and primary education or health care is that clinical research is only possible if some individuals bear certain risks—the risks of being research participants. In clinical research, unlike education or health care, to make gains for some persons, other persons experience risk of harm. Clinical research may help individuals experience a Rawlsian basic minimum or may help promote human capacities, but it comes at a cost of potential harm to participants. This is the justification for monitoring of clinical research: DSMBs are part of a system designed to manage those costs. Even if it were true that there is some basic minimum of the fruits of clinical research that all persons should be accorded, and that basic minimum is set by human capacities, those minimums are only achieved by putting other individuals at risk of harm in human studies.

Two conclusions emerge from this discussion. First, IA, although a coherent and attractive theory, may not be well suited to guide clinical research, a project that requires sacrifice on the part of some so as to promote the best outcome for the whole. Research on human beings involves maximizing the best outcome for individuals or groups—both of which involve welfarism and sum-ranking. Second, given the consequentialist nature of the research enterprise, independent monitoring is required to oversee clinical research to ensure that those consequences are, in fact, maximized as research unfolds. DSMBs are part of a complex monitoring system, including the input of sponsors, medical monitors, and IRBs. Significantly, DSMBs are necessary to oversee research as it begins in many cases, and always as it progresses, to ensure that the welfare of research participants and the sum-ranking of benefits over burdens remain intact.

A final note: Some utilitarians will take issue with the fact that London's view of utilitarianism is a bit narrow, failing to take into account recent advances in adjusting utilitarianism for concerns of justice and desert. Welfarism and sum-ranking may be necessary to a utilitarian ethic, but they may not be sufficient. In taking aim at a less sophisticated version of utilitarianism, contemporary utilitarians may argue, London is not entirely persuasive.

Equipoise, Anti-equipoise, and DSMBs

A second argument for the consequentialist nature of research ethics can be found in a response to the anti-equipoise theorists. Several bioethicists have come forward to challenge the orthodoxy on clinical equipoise, saying that it is not a necessary condition for ethical trials. Two claims made in the previous section, rejecting both the therapeutic stance of clinical research and the "best care" model, anticipated more detailed arguments discussed below by the anti-equipoise theorists. However, before examining their arguments, the arguments in favor of equipoise as an ethical requirement of clinical research should be briefly revisited.

Recall that in chapter 4, two types of arguments for the ethical necessity of equipoise were considered. The first type of argument was one that defends equipoise by saying that it is foundational to the methodology of clinical research. If one treatment is known to be better than another—if they are not in equipoise—then there is no point in starting a clinical trial to compare the two. If during the course of a trial, a study falls out of equipoise, and it is definitely demonstrated that one treatment arm is found to be better than another, then there is no point in continuing the trial. The very methodology of clinical research presupposes the centrality of equipoise. The second type of argument was one that proceeds from the "personal care" notion, that the duties of beneficence and nonmalefi-cence demand participants who have volunteered to be randomized into arms of a study deserve a promotion of benefit and avoidance of harm, if not for each participant individually, for the aggregate of research partici-pants in the study. Just as patients whose health is looked after by a physi-cian deserve to be treated with personal care, so too, research participants should be treated so that benefits are maximized and harm is diminished for the aggregate of participants as much as possible.

Litton and Miller are among those who don't subscribe to the notion that equipoise is central to the ethics of clinical research. They note with respect to Emanuel, Wendler, and Grady's seven requirements,

> Emanuel and colleagues assert that clinical equipoise is implied by their ethical framework. . . . It has been argued elsewhere that clinical equipoise confuses the ethics of clinical research with the ethical of medical care. We do not repeat the argument here but affirm the conclusion that clinical equipoise is not a necessary component of an ethical framework appropriate to clinical research. Therefore, it is important to recognize that our version of the ethical requirements on clinical research does not presuppose or imply clinical equipoise or any other version of equipoise. (Litton and Miller 2005, 569)

Arguments against the need for clinical equipoise, especially at the com-mencement of a study, look to concerns about paternalistic violations of autonomy or a misguided application of the therapeutic misconception. This is the ethic of personal care gone too far, precluding the "bad choice" study, not allowing for replication studies or other over-exacting limitations on clinical researchers.

Miller and Brody (2003) make a similar move when they dismiss equi-poise as a necessary condition for ethical research. Recall that Miller and Brody stated that the "similarity position," the view that ethics of clinical care and of research are similar, is mistaken. Instead, they hold that the ethics of clinical research is decidedly utilitarian. When examining Eman-uel, Wendler, and Grady's first and third requirements of ethical research (risks to participants must be reasonable; research must have social value), they contend that these are not the same as demonstrating a project is in equipoise. They embrace a non-exploitation framework (Joffe and Truog 2008) in which, as long as participants have offered informed consent, risks are minimized, and the research is of social benefit, then equipoise is not ethically necessary. The social benefit of the research needs to be maintained; the need for indifference among treatments for participants, investigators, or the clinical community does not.

A curious conclusion emerges from Brody and Miller's position. As long as participants who freely give informed consent aren't placed at undue risk and the research is of societal benefit, along with the other four of Emanuel, Wendler, and Grady's requirements, then the research is morally acceptable. *The research doesn't have to start in equipoise.* But as the research progresses, imagine that it becomes clear that one arm of the study is decidedly superior or inferior to the other. Or imagine that it becomes clear that the study is incapable of determining that one arm is decidedly superior or inferior to the other. Perhaps the study has reached a point of futility, for example, owing to a lack of recruitment (both conclusions, either that the study has prematurely achieved its outcome or is unable to achieve its outcome, are determinations first made by DSMBs). At that point, it is no longer of societal benefit for the research to continue, since the question as to which of the two arms is preferable has been answered or is incapable of being answered in that study. In other words, once the study is in progress, if it has been shown to not be of societal value to continue, then it is unethical. One way of failing to be of societal value is if the study is incapable of being completed for lack of retention, for example. But the other is if the study *in some sense has already been completed*—the study is no longer of societal value because the clinical question has already been answered. It has been convincingly demonstrated that one arm presents greater benefits or greater harms than the other. This is just another way of saying *the study is no longer in equipoise.* This is why monitoring studies is so crucial—once the DSMB reaches the conclusion that a study has answered its question or is incapable of answering the question it set out to answer, then the DSMB should recommend the study be stopped.

Although prominent bioethicists have made compelling arguments against a requirement of clinical equipoise at the beginning of a study, they have not made the case that a disruption of equipoise *during a study* is a similarly benign state of affairs. The need to maintain equipoise during the duration of a clinical protocol isn't attributable to a misguided paternalism or wrongheaded therapeutic misconception. The reason that equipoise is necessary during the course of the study is found in a methodological argument. What is the *point* of research but to reach a conclusion to advance generalizable knowledge? If a conclusion has been reached, a further demand on research participants is unnecessary. Recall the discussion in chapter 4—what it means for one arm to be clearly superior or inferior to another is complex, conceivably incorporating perspectives of research participants, investigators, and the clinical community. What it means for equipoise to be genuinely disrupted is not straightforward. However the fact that it is difficult to discern when equipoise has been disrupted does not detract from its centrality. A violation of equipoise at the commencement of a study, owing to the need for replication or other considerations, is arguably ethical. The consequentialist nature of clinical research is reaffirmed by the requirement of equipoise *during the execution of a study*, owing to the objectives of clinical research.

Given the two-pronged argument for the claim that clinical research is a consequentialist enterprise—the negative argument against principlism and the positive argument in favor of consequentialism—it follows that the ethical scrutiny of clinical research isn't a one-time proposition. The bulk of scrutiny shouldn't happen before a study commences, as is done by IRBs. IRBs have an important role in maintaining ethical engagement with research participants. But the greater ethical engagement emerges over the course of trials, the point at which DSMBs take over. Research projects should be evaluated throughout their duration to ensure that participants remain informed, to determine that if risks change their continued participation is justified, and to monitor equipoise.

Conclusion

What lessons can be learned from the above discussion? First, it is my contention that clinical research is guided by a consequentialist ethic. As such, the guiding question determining if a research study is ethical is whether the consequences—for the researchers, the research participants, and those who will benefit from the research—will be the best possible. The consequences for all parties matter, and the consequences during all points in the design and execution of the study matter. If at any point in the study, the risks of harm to participants outweigh the potential benefits of the research, benefits to both current participants *and* future cohorts, then the study is no longer ethical. Although it is important to obtain voluntary informed consent when at all possible and maintain a just selection of participants, placing an undue emphasis on examination of a research study *before it even begins* is not being true to the consequentialist ethic guiding human research.

Although the work of the DSMB is in part focused on the design of the study, or the crafting of sound informed consent documents before the study begins, these are only the first steps in ethically sound research. Continual monitoring of the study, to ensure that at every juncture, the consequences of the study are the best they can be, is the ongoing work of the DSMB. As shown in chapter 1, the IRB system was designed primarily to assess projects before they begin, with comparatively little emphasis on continuing review of protocols in progress. This isn't surprising, given that the Common Rule and the *Belmont Report* were borne from scandals surrounding research that *should never have commenced in the first place*. With the recognition of the consequentialist nature of research comes a recognition that the bulk of ethical assessment of research takes place after the research commences. DSMB's primary emphasis is on trials while they are in progress, to make sure that the potential benefits continue to outweigh the potential risks.

DSMB work is among the most challenging and meaningful work I've done as a bioethicist. In this book, I've shown the uniquely valuable perspective that ethicists bring to DSMB work, demonstrated how NIH-sponsored trials I've helped to monitor illuminate important lessons for those engaged in DSMB work, and examined the theoretical foundations that inform DSMB deliberations. While serving on DSMBs, my role was to collaborate with statisticians and clinicians to help keep participants safe. Clinical research is a high-risk and high-reward enterprise, and the participants who take the risks aren't always the ones who reap the rewards. My hope is that this volume assists those who play a part in giving voice to those participants.

Notes

Introduction

1. Throughout, I will be adopting the contemporary nomenclature, referring to individuals on who volunteer to serve in clinical studies as "participants." Elsewhere in the literature, they are also referred to as "subjects." As Capron notes, however, "As a general matter, dressing 'subjects' up as 'participants' may just lessen the felt need to prevent their suffering avoidable harm and violation of rights" (Capron 2014, 151).

2. For those interested in the statistical analysis employed by DSMBs, excellent resources include *Data Monitoring in Clinical Trials: A Case Studies Approach*, edited by David L. DeMets, Curt D. Furberg, and Lawrence M. Friedman (Springer, 2006); *Statistical Monitoring of Clinical Trials: A Unified Approach* by Michael A. Proschan, K. K. Gordon Lan, and Janet Turk Wittles (Springer, 2006); and *Data Monitoring Committees in Clinical Trials: A Practical Perspective* by Susan S. Ellenberg, Thomas R. Fleming, and David L. DeMets (John Wiley & Sons, 2019). Jay Herson's *Data and Safety Monitoring in Clinical Trials*, 2nd edition (Taylor and Francis, 2017) is both a rigorous and approachable guide that includes helpful Q&As at the end of each chapter for members of monitoring committees. Paul G. Wakim and Pamela A. Shaw's chapter "Data and Safety Monitoring" in *Principles and Practice of Clinical Research*, 4th edition (ed. Gallin, Ognibene, and Johnson, Academic Press, 2018) is a concise but comprehensive resource on the procedural aspects of DSMBs.

3. How much more familiar? In a search of the Philosopher's Index on January 19, 2022, there were 173 results for the "subject" search of "IRB or Institutional Review Board." A "subject" search of "DSMB or DSMC or data monitoring" yielded 3 results.

4. See "Revised Common Rule," accessed October 10, 2024, https://www.hhs.gov/ohrp/regulations-and-policy/regulations/finalized-revisions-common-rule/index.html.

5. Per the DAMOCLES study group, "We propose that groups responsible for data monitoring be given the standard name, Data Monitoring Committee (DMC)" (2005, 711).

6. A similar approach, discussing the issues that emerge when engaging in DSMB oversight while not betraying specific confidential discussions, can be found in Wittes et al. (2007); see also Canner (1983) and DeMets, Furberg, and Friedman (2006).

1 What Are Data Safety Monitoring Boards, and What Is Their Role?

1. See, for example, Rebecca Dresser's candid description of her reluctance to join a clinical trial (Dresser 2012, 74): "Of course, I was not the typical patient invited to join a study. Instead, I was quite familiar with how trials worked. For many years, I had served on my school's Institutional Review Board (IRB), the committee that evaluates research proposals to ensure that they meet ethical and regulatory standards."

2. A list of the twenty Federal Agencies that follow Common Rule Guidance, and the details of their engagement, can be found at "Federal Policy for the Protection of Human Subjects ('Common Rule')," U.S. Department of Health and Human Services, accessed October 10, 2022, https://www.hhs.gov/ohrp/regulations-and-policy /regulations/common-rule/index.html#:~:text=The%20Federal%20Policy%20for%20 the,and%20agencies%2C%20as%20listed%20below.

3. It can be argued that the Tuskegee study, unethical at its inception, became *even more unethical* as time went on. Once penicillin was discovered as a treatment for syphilis and put into widespread production and use, the study was even less justified. At the point that a cure was found, the justification for continuing to monitor men with a terminal and contagious disease became even more heinous than it was at the study's initiation. The fact that penicillin was discovered as a treatment for syphilis during the course of the study doesn't ethically justify the study at its inception, however.

4. See "Guidance for Industry: Using a Centralized IRB Review Process in Multi-center Clinical Trials," FDA, accessed July 25, 2023, https://www.fda.gov/media /75329/download.

2 What Does an Ethicist Bring to the DSMB? The STRIVE- IPF Trial

1. One "strategy for minimizing the number of subjects exposed to the inferior intervention involves unbalanced randomization, with a ratio favoring the preferred arm" (Joffe and Truog 2008, 251). This is a controversial strategy, as some argue it is not statistically efficient, per an anonymous reviewer of this manuscript.

2. "Autoantibody Reduction for Acute Exacerbations of Idiopathic Pulmonary Fibrosis (STRIVE-IPF)," NIH National Library of Medicine, accessed September 27, 2024, https://clinicaltrials.gov/ct2/show/NCT03286556.

3. "Healthcare Ethics Consultant-Certified Program," HEC-C, accessed September 27, 2024, https://heccertification.org/.

4. That being said, the STRIVE-IPF consent form was nonetheless extremely long, given the numerous tests, procedures, and uncertainties of this phase II trial. Long consent forms persist as the norm (Appelbaum and Lidz 2008). See, for example, Emanuel and Boyle (2021), whose analysis of informed consent documents for four phase III COVID-19 vaccine trials found the consent forms were a mean of 21.8 pages long, with a range of 17 to 25 pages.

5. "Harm" in research shouldn't be restricted to physical harms. Per the Common Rule, "minimal risk" research is that for which the harms and discomforts "are not greater in and of themselves than those ordinarily encountered in everyday life or during the performance of routine physical or psychological tests" (§46.102(7j)), which may include anxiety, frustration, boredom, and the like. The Common Rule recognizes breach of confidentiality as a harm. The harms of the Humphrey visual field test may not be physical, but are no less real.

6. This is reminiscent of a point made by Dresser (2017, 49), that annual memory tests by healthy participants in an Alzheimer's study might seem low risk but can be stressful to participants because of anxiety surrounding their performance.

7. "Autoantibody Reduction for Acute Exacerbations of Idiopathic Pulmonary Fibrosis (STRIVE-IPF)," NIH National Library of Medicine, accessed September 27, 2024, https://clinicaltrials.gov/ct2/show/study/NCT03286556#contacts. As with many clinical trials that were initiated before 2020 and were scheduled to run through 2020, this study was extended due to the pandemic.

8. A full discussion of the DSMB's role in evaluating AE's is discussed in chapter 3.

9. "Reviewing and Reporting Unanticipated Problems Involving Risks to Subjects or Others and Adverse Events: OHRP Guidance (2007)," U.S. Department of Health and Human Services, accessed September 27, 2024, https://www.hhs.gov/ohrp/regulations-and-policy/guidance/reviewing-unanticipated-problems/index.html#Q2.

10. I thank an anonymous reviewer for stressing this point.

3 Measuring Risks, Informing Participants: The CALEC Trial

1. See "Information for Potential Patients," JCHR, accessed September 27, 2024, https://public.jaeb.org/calec/view/PotentialPatients as well as "Limbal Stem Cell Deficiency (LSCD) Treatment with Cultivated Stem Cell (CALEC) Graft (CALEC)," NIH National Library of Medicine, accessed September 27, 2024, https://www.clinicaltrials.gov/study/NCT02592330. I say that the study "began" as a comparison between CALEC and CLAU because owing to complex factors, the study was unable to continue as initially conceived and was ultimately reconfigured as an uncontrolled study of CALEC. The discussion of the CALEC trial presented here, which focuses on DSMB discussions prior to initiation of the study, reflects the study as initially conceived.

2. Despite being uttered years ago, those nine words haunted me. They made it clear just how much was at stake in the CALEC and CLAU procedures.

3. I wish to thank an anonymous reviewer for urging this point be made explicit.

4. For an interesting discussion arguing against the use of research resources to fund trials of new antibiotics, see Spencer Phillips Hey and Aaron S. Kesselheim's 2017 article "Reprioritizing Research Activity for the Post-antibiotic Era: Ethical, Legal and Social Considerations," *Hastings Center Report* 47(2) (March): 16–20.

5. One of the complexities in making an assessment about potential risks and benefits of a study drug is that whether the drug or intervention in the study is reasonably expected to have caused an AE can be a matter of individual clinician judgment. All AEs are reported, and many are based on objective criteria (did the participant have a rash or not? Did the participant experience a fever?). However, whether the AE was *reasonably caused by the intervention* can be a judgment call on the part of the individual clinician. There may be cases in which clinicians judge that the intervention likely didn't cause the AE, and only after examining the aggregate data is it clear that a trend emerges signaling the AEs may have resulted from the investigatory drug or article. For this reason, the below table doesn't portray the incidence of a rash as zero, even at the twenty-four-week mark. It is possible—even likely—that some participants will have a rash at twenty-four weeks, even if it isn't reasonably expected to have been caused by the experimental antibiotic.

4 Equipoise and Stopping Studies: Protocols AG and AH

1. Another significant concern in the SUPPORT trial included perceived inadequacies of the consent forms (Grady 2015).

2. For more on the debate on the SUPPORT study, see Defino (2014).

3. The precise definition of *equipoise* is so disputed that Joffe and Troug (2008), as well as Veatch (2009), prefer to use the term "indifference."

4. Those people turned out to be wrong.

5. In ophthalmology studies such as protocols AG and AH, the CALEC study discussed in chapter 3, and the SIGHT trial discussed in chapter 5, the convention is to use the terms "masked" or "double masked" when referring to the state of affairs in which participants, or participants and investigators, respectively, are not told into which arm the participant has been randomized. Elsewhere, such as when discussing the STRIVE-IPF study, I use the widely used convention of referring to these as "blind" or "double blind" studies. Herson (2017) uses the term "masked."

6. The question as to whether the AEs should have been pooled across both studies, or grouped separately in the AG and AH studies, may occur to some. Wittes et al. (2007), in discussing the Women's Health Initiative clinical trials, recount that the

DSMB was charged with overseeing both the PERT trial (estrogen plus progestin) and the ERT trial (estrogen alone) for postmenopausal women. The question as to whether the data should have been pooled in the PERT and ERT trials wasn't clear-cut: on one hand, "separating the data from the two trials would produce underestimates of the strength of the evidence for harm or benefit (2017, 223)," but on the other hand, some data emerged that pulled in the opposite direction.

7. For reference, in my state of Ohio, a person with vision 20/40 or better is legally permitted to get a driver's license without corrective lenses such as glasses or contacts. With corrected vision at 20/60 in one eye, a person is permitted a driver's license. See "Ohio Laws & Administrative Rules: Vision Standards for Driver License Applicants," accessed October 10, 2024, https://codes.ohio.gov/ohio-administrative -code/rule-4501:1-1-20.

5 Recruitment, Retention, and Keeping Vulnerable Participants Safe: The SIGHT Trial

1. Portions of this chapter were published earlier in Deborah R. Barnbaum, 2020, "Data safety monitoring during COVID-19: Keep on keeping on," *Ethics & Human Research* 42(3) (May–June): 43–44.

2. "Surgical Idiopathic Intracranial Hypertension Treatment Trial (SIGHT)," NIH National Library of Medicine, accessed September 27, 2024, https://clinicaltrials .gov/ct2/show/NCT03501966?term=SIGHT&recrs=eghim&cond=Idiopathic+Intracr anial+Hypertension&cntry=US&draw=2&rank=1.

3. I thank an anonymous reviewer for this important example.

4. The NIH took note of this fact and mandated all protocols follow NIH Notice NOT-OD-20-087, "Guidance for NIH-funded Clinical Trials and Human Subjects Studies Affected by COVID-19," https://grants.nih.gov/grants/guide/notice-files/NOT-OD-20 -087.html.

5. The following discussion concerns studies that were initiated before the pandemic began and thus were not conceived with the intention to study COVID-19, its vaccines, or treatment. For a discussion of the role of DSMBs in studies initiated to study COVID, see Eckstein et al. (2021).

6. This important point was articulated by an anonymous reviewer.

7. I thank Janet Wittes for making this point.

6 The Theoretical Foundations of DSMB Deliberations

1. J. L. Austin, *Philosophical Papers*, 1979, eds. James Opie and Geoffrey James Warnock, 3rd ed. New York: Oxford, 185: "Ordinary language is *not* the last word: in

principle it can everywhere be supplemented and improved upon and superseded. Only remember, it is the *first* word."

2. The additional protections afforded to prisoners, outlined in the Common Rule part C, are also the result of decades of abuse of prisoners by researchers, owing to their diminished autonomy. Thus, part C is not merely about an acknowledgment of the compromised nature of prison life, but the historical injustices perpetated against prisoners. For a discussion of the missed opportunities when revising the Common Rule for extending greater protections to prisoners who serve in research, see Obasogie (2014).

References

Abbott, Lura, and Christine Grady. 2011. "A systematic review of the empirical literature evaluating IRBs: What we know and what we still need to learn." *Journal of Empirical Human Research Ethics* 6(1) (March): 3–19.

Acuna, Sergio A., Tyler R. Chesney, and Nancy N. Baxter. 2019. "Incorporating patient preferences into noninferiority trials." *Journal of the American Medical Association* 322(4) (July 23): 305–306.

Age-Related Eye Disease Study Group. 1999. "Design implications AREDS report no. 1." *Controlled Clinical Trials* 20(6) (December): 573–600.

Age-Related Eye Disease Study Research Group. 2001. "A randomized, placebo-controlled, clinical trial of high-dose supplementation with vitamins C and E, beta carotene, and zinc for age-related macular degeneration and vision loss: AREDS report no. 8." *Archive of Ophthalmology* 119(10) (October):1417–1436.

Alpha-Tocopherol, Beta-Carotene Cancer Prevention Study Group. 1994. The effect of vitamin E and beta carotene on the incidence of lung cancer and other cancers in male smokers. *New England Journal of Medicine* 330(15) (April 14): 1029–1035.

Angus, Derek C., Anthony C. Gordon, and Howard Bauchner. 2021. "Emerging lessons from COVID-19 for the US clinical research enterprise." *Journal of the American Medical Association* 325(12) (March 23): 1159–1161.

Appelbaum, Paul S., and Charles W. Lidz. 2008. "The therapeutic misconception." In *The Oxford Textbook of Clinical Research Ethics*, edited by Ezikiel Emanuel, Christine Grady, Robert A. Crouch, Reidar K. Lie, Franklin G. Miller, and David Wendler, 633–644. New York: Oxford University Press.

Barnbaum, Deborah R. 2019. "Randomization among: The other randomization." *Ethics & Human Research* 41(5) (September–October): 35–40.

Barnbaum, Deborah R. 2020. "Data safety monitoring during COVID-19: Keep on keeping on." *Ethics & Human Research* 42(3) (May–June): 43–44.

Beauchamp, Tom L., and James F. Childress. 2019. *Principles of Biomedical Ethics*. 8th ed. New York: Oxford University Press.

Beecher, Henry K. 1966. "Ethics and clinical research." *New England Journal of Medicine* 274(24) (June 16): 1354–1360.

Berkman, Benjamin E., Dana Howard, and David Wendler. 2018. "Reconsidering the need for reconsent at 18." *Pediatrics* 142(2) (August): 1–5. https://doi.org/10.1542/peds.2017-1202.

Bibbins-Domingo, Kirsten, Alex Helman, and Victor Dzau. 2022. "The imperative for diversity and inclusion in clinical trials and health research participation." *Journal of the American Medical Association* 327(23) (June 21): 2283–2284.

Biddle, Justin. 2007. "Lessons from the Vioxx debacle: What the privatization of science can teach us about social epistemology." *Social Epistemology* 21(1) (January–March): 21–39.

Briggs, Ryan. 2022. "The abject failure of IRBs." *Chronicle of Higher Education*, March 23, 2022. https://www.chronicle.com/article/the-abject-failure-of-irbs.

Blumenthal, David, and Cara James. 2022. "A data infrastructure for clinical trial diversity." *New England Journal of Medicine* 386(25) (June 23): 2355–2356.

Bonham, Valerie, and Jonathan Moreno. 2008. "Research with captive populations: Prisoners, students, and soldiers." In *The Oxford Textbook of Clinical Research Ethics*, edited by Ezekiel Emanuel, Christine Grady, Robert A. Crouch, Reidar K. Lie, Franklin G. Miller, and David Wendler, 461–474. New York: Oxford University Press.

Borgerson, Kirstin. 2016. "An argument for fewer clinical trials." *Hastings Center Report* 46(6) (November–December): 25–35.

Bothwell, Laura E., and Aaron S. Kesselheim. 2017. "The real-world ethics of adaptive-design clinical trials." *Hastings Center Report* 47(6) (November–December): 27–37

Boyter, Elizabeth. 2019. "Idiopathic intracranial hypertension." *Journal of the American Academy of Physician Assistants* 32(5) (May): 30–35.

Braddock, Adam. 2014. "Children as research partners in community pediatrics." In *Human Subjects Research Regulation: Perspectives on the Future*, edited by I. Glenn Cohen and Holly Fernandez Lynch, 79–92. Cambridge, MA: MIT Press.

Brock, Dan W. 2008. "Philosophical justifications of informed consent in research." In *The Oxford Textbook of Clinical Research Ethics*, edited by Ezekiel Emanuel, Christine Grady, Robert A. Crouch, Reidar K. Lie, Franklin G. Miller, and David Wendler, 606–612. New York: Oxford University Press.

Brody, Baruch A., Laurence P. McCullough, and Richard R. Sharp. 2005. "Consensus and controversy in clinical research ethics." *Journal of the American Medical Association* 294(11) (September 21): 1411–1414.

Brown, Nancy C., and Summer Johnson McGee. 2014. "Conceptualizing boundaries for the professionalization of healthcare ethics practice: A call for empirical research." *HEC Forum* 26 (December): 325–341.

Cairns, John A., Alfred Hallstrom, and Peter Held. 2001. "Should all trials have a data safety and monitoring committee?" *American Heart Journal* 141(1) (January): 156–163.

Calis, Karim A., Patrick Archdeacon, Raymond P. Bain, Annemarie Forrest, Jane Perlmutter, and David L. DeMets. 2017. "Understanding the functions and operations of data monitoring committees: Survey and focus group findings." *Clinical Trials* 14(1) (February): 59–66.

Canner, Paul L. 1983. "Monitoring of the data for evidence of adverse or beneficial treatment effects." *Controlled Clinical Trials* 4(4) (December): 467–483.

Capron, Alexander Morgan. 2014. "Subjects, participants, and partners: What are the implications for research as the role of informed consent evolves?" In *Human Subjects Research Regulation: Perspectives on the Future*, edited by I. Glenn Cohen and Holly Fernandez Lynch, 143–155. Cambridge, MA: MIT Press.

Catania, Joseph A., Bernard Lo, Leslie E. Wolf, M. Margaret Dolcini, Lance M. Pollack, Judith C. Barker, Stacey Wertlieb, and Jeff Henne. 2008. "Survey of U.S. human research protection organizations: Workload and membership." *Journal of Empirical Research on Human Research Ethics* 3(4) (December): 57–69.

Char, Clement K., Calvin E. Mein, Adam R. Glassman, Wesley T. Beaulieu, Claire T. Calhoun, Glenn J. Jaffe, Lee M. Jampol, et al. 2021. "Pneumonic vitreolysis with perfluoropropane for vitreomacular traction with and without macular hole: DRCR retina network protocols AG and AH." *American Academy of Ophthalmology* 128(11) (November): 1592–1603.

Chidwick, Paula, Jennifer Bell, Eoin Connolly, Michael D. Coughlin, Andrea Frolic, Laurie Hardingham, and Randi Zlotnik Shaul. 2010. "Exploring a role model description for ethicists." *HEC Forum* 22 (March): 31–40.

Collins, Joseph F. 2003. "Data and safety monitoring board issues raised in the VA status epilepticus study." *Controlled Clinical Trials* 24(1) (February): 71–77.

Cummings, Steven R., and Michael C. Rowbotham. 2017. "Informed consent and internet-based trials." *New England Journal of Medicine* 376(9) (March 2): 859–861.

DAMOCLES Study Group. 2005. "A proposed charter for clinical trial data monitoring committees: Helping them to do their job well." *Lancet* 365(9460) (February): 711–722.

Davies, Ben. 2019. "Bursting bubbles? QALYs and discrimination." *Utilitas: A Journal of Utilitarian Studies* 31(2) (June): 191–202.

Davis, Amy L., and Elisa A. Hurley. 2014. "Setting the stage: The past and present of human subjects research regulation." In *Human Subjects Research Regulation Perspectives on the Future*, edited by I. Glenn Cohen and Holly Fernandez Lynch, 9–24. Cambridge, MA: MIT Press.

Defino, Theresa. 2014. "With just one investigation in 2013, OHRP seems 'Invisible' after SUPPORT dust-up." *Report on Research Compliance*. Accessed April 19, 2024. https://www.bmj.com/sites/default/files/response_attachments/2014/07/rrc-reprint -0514.pdf.

DeMets, David L., and Susan S. Ellenberg. 2016. "Data monitoring committees—Expect the unexpected." *New England Journal of Medicine* 375(14): 1365–1371.

DeMets, David L., Thomas R. Fleming, Frank Rockhold, Barry Massie, Thomas Merchant, Alan Meisel, Barbara Mishkin, Janet Wittes, David Stump, and Robert Califf. 2004. "Liability issues for data monitoring committee members." *Clinical Trials* 1(6): 525–531.

DeMets, David L., and Lawrence M. Friedman. 2006. "The data monitoring experience in the cardiac arrhythmia suppression trial: The need to be prepared early." In *Data Monitoring in Clinical Trials: A Case Studies Approach*, edited by David L. DeMets, Curt D. Furberg, and Lawrence M. Friedman, 198–208. New York: Springer.

DeMets, David L, Curt D. Furberg, and Lawrence M. Friedman, eds. 2006. *Data Monitoring in Clinical Trials: A Case Studies Approach*. New York: Springer.

Department of Health and Human Services, Office of the Inspector General. 2013. Data safety monitoring boards in NIH clinical trials: Meeting guidance, but facing some issues. OEI-12-11-00070 (June).

Department of Health and Human Services, Office of the Secretary. 2011. "Human subjects research protections: Enhancing protections for human research subjects and reducing burden, delay, and ambiguity for investigators." *Federal Register* 76(143) (July 26): 44512–44531.

Dresser, Rebecca. 2008. "The role of patient advocates and public representatives in research." In *The Oxford Textbook of Clinical Research Ethics*, edited by Ezekiel J. Emanuel, Christine Grady, Robert A. Crouch, Reidar K. Lie, Franklin G. Miller, and David Wendler, 231–241. New York: Oxford University Press.

Dresser, Rebecca. 2012. "Volunteering for research." In *Malignant: Medical Ethicists Confront Cancer*, edited by Rebecca Dresser, 70–85. New York: Oxford University Press.

Dresser, Rebecca. 2017. *Silent Partners: Human Subjects and Research Ethics*. New York: Oxford University Press.

Eckstein, Lisa. 2015. "Building a more connected DSMB: Better integrating ethics review and safety monitoring." *Accountability in Research* 22(2): 81–105.

Eckstein, Lisa, Annette Rid, Docras Kamuya, and Seema K. Shah. 2021. "The essential role of data safety monitoring boards (DSMBs) in ensuring the ethics of global vaccine trials to address coronavirus disease 2019 (COVID-19)." *Clinical Infectious Diseases* 73(11) (December): 2126–2130.

Ellenberg, Susan S., Thomas R. Fleming, and David L. DeMets. 2019. *Monitoring Committees in Clinical Trials: A Practical Perspective.* 2nd ed. Hoboken, NJ: John Wiley & Son.

EMA, CHMP (European Medicines Agency/Committee for Medicinal Products for Human Use). 2005. "Guideline on data monitoring committees." Accessed April 20, 2024. https://ema.europa.eu/en/documents/scientific-guideline/guideline-data -monitoring-committees_en.pdf.

Emanuel, Ezekiel J. 2014. "Why I hope to die at 75." *The Atlantic.* Accessed April 20, 2024. https://www.theatlantic.com/magazine/archive/2014/10/why-i-hope-to-die-at -75/379329/.

Emanuel, Ezekiel J., and Conner W. Boyer. 2021. "Assessment of length and readability of informed consent documents for COVID-19 vaccine trials." *JAMA Network Open* 4(4): 1–5. Accessed January 28, 2022. https://jamanetwork.com/journals /jamanetworkopen/fullarticle/2779247.

Emanuel, Ezekiel J., and Jerry Menikoff. 2011. "Reforming the regulations governing research with human subjects." *New England Journal of Medicine* 365(12) (September 22 : 1145–1150.

Emanuel, Ezekiel J., David Wendler, and Christine Grady. 2000. "What makes clinical research ethical?" *Journal of the American Medical Association* 283(20) (May): 2701–2711.

Fader, Ruth, Nancy Kass, Danielle Whicher, Walter Stewart, and Sean Tunis. 2013. "Ethics and informed consent for comparative effectiveness research with prospective electronic clinical data." *Medical Care* 51(8, Suppl 3): 553–557.

Feldman, Heidi Li. 2014. "What's right about the medical model in human subjects research regulation." In *Human Subjects Research Regulation: Perspectives on the Future,* edited by I. Glenn Cohen and Holly Fernandez Lynch, 299–311. Cambridge, MA: MIT Press.

Fernandez Lynch, Holly, Thomas C. Darton, Jae Levy, Frank McCormick, Ubaka Ogbogu, Ruth O. Payne, Alvin E. Roth, Akilah Jefferson Shah, Thomas Smiley, and Emily A. Largent. 2021. "Promoting ethical payment in human infection challenge studies." *American Journal of Bioethics* 21(3) (March): 11–31.

Fernandez Lynch, Holly, Elisa A. Hurley, and Holly A. Taylor. 2023. "Responding to the call to meaningfully assess Institutional Review Board effectiveness." *JAMA* 330(3 (June 23): 221–222.

Floyd, Anna, and Anne Moyer. 2010. "Effects of participant preferences in unbl nded randomized controlled trials." *Journal of Empirical Research on Human Research Ethics* 5(2) (June): 81–93.

Franklin, Donald. 2017. "Calibrating QALYs to respect equality of persons." *U ilitas: A Journal of Utilitarian Studies* 29(1): 65–87.

Freedman, Benjamin. 1987. "Equipoise and the ethics of clinical research." *New England Journal of Medicine* 317(3) (July): 141–145.

Fried, Charles. 2016. *Medical Experimentation: Personal Integrity and Social olicy.* Edited by Franklin Miller and Alan Wertheimer. New York: Oxford University ress.

Friedman, Lawrence M., and Eleanor B. Schron. 2008. "Data and safety manitoring boards." In *The Oxford Textbook of Clinical Research Ethics*, edited by Ezekiel J. Emanuel, Christine Grady, Robert A. Crouch, Reidar K. Lie, Franklin G. Miller, and David Wendler, 569–576. New York: Oxford University Press.

GAO-23-104721. 2023. "Institutional review boards: Actions needed to improve federal oversight and examine effectiveness." Accessed May 26, 2023. https://gao .gov/products/gao-23-104721#:~:text=FDA%20and%20HHS's%20Office%20 for,routine%20or%20for%2Dcause%20inspections.

Gelinas, Luke, Alan Wertheimer, and Franklin G. Miller. 2016. "When and why is research without consent permissible?" *Hastings Center Report* 46(2) (March–April): 35–43.

Gifford, Fred. 2007. "So-called 'clinical equipoise' and the argument from design." *Journal of Medicine and Philosophy* 32(2) (March–April): 135–150.

Gordon, Valery M., Jeremy Sugarman, and Nancy Kass. 1998. "Toward a more comprehensive approach to protecting human subjects: The interface of Data Safety Monitoring Boards and Institutional Review Boards in randomized clinical trials." *IRB: A Review of Human Subjects Research* 20(1) (January–February): 1–5.

Grady, Christine. 2015. "Enduring and emerging challenges of informed consent." *New England Journal of Medicine* 372(9) (February 26): 855–860.

Grady, Christine. 2017. "The changing face of informed consent." *New England Journal of Medicine* 376(9) (March 2): 856–859.

Grady, Christine. 2019. "Bioethics in the oversight of clinical research: Institutional Review Boards and Data Safety Monitoring Boards." *Kennedy Institute of Ethics Journal* 29(1) (March): 33–49.

Heart Special Project Committee to the National Advisory Heart Council. 1988. "Organization, review, and administration of cooperative studies (Greenberg Report)." *Controlled Clinical Trials* 9(2) (June): 137–148.

Hellman, Samuel, and Deborah S. Hellman. 1991. "Of mice but not men—Problems of the randomized clinical trial." *New England Journal of Medicine* 324(2) (May 30): 1585–1589.

Hennekens, Charles H., Julie E. Buring, JoAnn E. Manson, Meir Stampfer, Bernard Rosner, Nancy R. Cook, Charlene Belanger, et al. 1996. "Lack of effect of long-term supplementation with beta carotene on the incidence of malignant neoplasms and cardiovascular disease." *New England Journal of Medicine* 334(1) (May 2): 1145–1149.

Herson, Jay. 2017. *Data and Safety Monitoring Committees in Clinical Trials.* 2nd ed. Boca Raton, FL: CRC Press.

Hey, Spencer Phillips, and Aaron S. Kesselheim. 2017. "Reprioritizing research activity for the post-antibiotic era: Ethical, legal and social considerations." *Hastings Center Report* 47(2) (March): 16–20.

Hillary, Frank G., and John D. Medaglia. 2020. "What the replication crisis means for intervention science." *International Journal of Psychophysiology* 154 (August): 3–5.

Horng, Sam, and Christine Grady. 2003. "Misunderstanding in clinical research: Distinguishing the therapeutic misconception, therapeutic misestimation, and therapeutic optimism." *IRB: Ethics & Human Research* 25(1) (January–February): 11–16.

Hudson, Kathy L., Alan E. Guttmacher, and Francis S. Collins. 2013. "In support of SUPPORT—A view from the NIH." *New England Journal of Medicine* 368(25) (June 20): 2349–2351.

Jamrozik, Euzebiusz, and Michael J. Selgelid. 2020. "Ethical issues surrounding controlled human infection challenge studies in endemic low- and middle-income countries." *Bioethics* 34(8) (October): 797–808.

Janevic, Mary, Nancy K. Janz, Julia A. Dodge, Xihong Lin, Wenqin Pan, Brandy R. Sinco, and Noreen M. Clark. 2003. "The role of choice in health education intervention trials: A review and case study." *Social Science and Medicine* 56(2) (April): 1581–1594.

Jansen, Lynn A., Paul S. Appelbaum, William M. P. Klein, Neil D. Weinstein, William Cook, Jessica S. Fogel, and Daniel P. Sulmasy. 2011. "Unrealistic optimism in early phase oncology trials." *IRB: Ethics & Human Research* 33(1) (January–February): 1–8.

Joffe, Steven, and Robert D. Truog. 2008. "Equipoise and randomization." In *The Oxford Textbook of Clinical Research Ethics*, edited by Ezekiel J. Emanuel, Christine Grady, Robert A. Crouch, Reidar K. Lie, Franklin G. Miller, and David Wendler, 245–260. New York: Oxford University Press.

Jurkunas, Ula, Lynette Johns, and Myriam Armant. 2022. "Cultivated autologous limbal epithelial cell transplantation: New frontier in the treatment of limbal stem cell deficiency." *American Journal of Ophthalmology* 239 (July): 244–268.

Kang, Gagandeep, 2017. "Video informed consent." *New England Journal of Medicine* 376(9) (March 2): 863–867.

Kerr, David, and Nand Kishore Rawat, eds. 2023. *Data Monitoring Committees (DMCs): Past, Present, and Future*. Cham, Switzerland: Springer ebook. https://doi.org/10.1007/978-3-031-28760-2.

Kim, Tae Jun, and Olaf von dem Knesebeck. 2018. "Income and obesity: What is the direction of the relationship? A systematic review and meta-analysis." *British Medical Journal Open* 8(1) (January 5): 1–13.

Klein, Lauren, Joanna Moore, and Michelle Biros. 2018. "A 20-year review: The use of exception from informed consent and waiver of informed consent in emergency research." *Academic Emergency Medicine* 25(10) (October): 1081–1188.

Klitzman, Robert. 2015. *The Ethics Police? The Struggle to Make Human Research Safe*. New York: Oxford University Press.

Koski, Greg. 2014. "Getting past protectionism: Is it time to take off the training wheels?" In *Human Subjects Research Regulation: Perspectives on the Future*, edited by I. Glenn Cohen and Holly Fernandez Lynch, 340–348. Cambridge, MA: MIT University Press.

Krumholz, Harlan, Joseph S. Ross, Amos H. Presler, and David S. Egilman. 2007. "What have we learnt from Vioxx?" *British Medical Journal* 334(7585) (January 20): 120–123.

Lantos, John D., and Chris Feudtner. 2015. "SUPPORT and the ethics of study implementation: Lessons for comparative effectiveness research from the trial of oxygen therapy for premature babies." *Hastings Center Report* 45(1) (January–February): 30–40.

Largent, Emily A., Holly Fernandez Lynch, and Matthew S. McCoy. 2018. "Patient-engaged research: Choosing the 'right' patients to avoid pitfalls." *Hastings Center Report* 48(5) (September–October): 26–34.

Ledford, Heidi. 2020. "Coronavirus shuts down trials of drugs for multiple other diseases." *Nature* 580(7801) (April 2): 15–16.

Levine, Carol. 1988. "Has AIDS changed the ethics of human subjects research?" *Journal of Law, Medicine, and Ethics* 16(3–4) (Fall–Winter): 167–173.

Litton, Paul, and Franklin G. Miller. 2005. "A normative justification for distinguishing the ethics of clinical research from the ethics of medical care." *Journal of Law, Medicine & Ethics* 33(3) (Fall): 566–574.

Lo, Bernard. 2003. "Deciding for patients who have lost their decision-making capacity—Finding common ground in medical ethics." *New England Journal of Medicine* 389(25) (December 21): 2309–2312.

London, Alex John. 2007a. "Clinical equipoise: Foundational requirement or fundamental error?" In *The Oxford Handbook of Bioethics*, edited by Bonnie Steinbock, 571–596. New York: Oxford University Press.

London, Alex John. 2007b. "Two dogmas of research ethics and the integrative approach to human-subjects research." *Journal of Medicine and Philosophy* 32(2) (March–April): 99–116.

London, Alex John, and Jonathan Kimmelman. 2019. "Clinical trial portfolios: A critical oversight in human research ethics, drug regulation, and policy." *Hastings Center Report* 49(4) (July–August): 31–41.

Lou, Qiankun, and Tao Qin. 2020. "Managing clinical trials for COVID-19: The importance of ethics committees." *British Medical Journal* 369 (April 3): m1369.

Lynch, John. 2011. "'Through a glass darkly': Researcher ethnocentrism and the demonization of research participants." *American Journal of Bioethics* 11(4) (April): 22–23.

Mansbach, Jonathan, Uchechi Acholonu, Sunday Clark, and Carlos A. Camargo, Jr. 2007. "Variation in Institutional Review Board responses to a standard, observational, pediatric research protocol." *Academic Emergency Medicine* 14(4) (April): 377–380.

Maschke, Karen J., and Michael K. Gusmano. 2020. "Ethics and evidence in the search for a vaccine and treatments for COVID-19." *Hastings Bioethics Forum*. Accessed April 21, 2024. https://www.thehastingscenter.org/ethics-and-evidence-in -the-search-for-a-vaccine-and-treatments-for-COVID-19/.

McConnell, Michael V., and Euan A. Ashley. 2017. "Mobile health research— App-based trials and informed consent." *New England Journal of Medicine* 376(9) (March 2): 861–863.

Meinert, Curtis L. 1998. "Masked monitoring in clinical trials—Blind stupidity?" *New England Journal of Medicine* 388(19) (May 17): 1381–1382.

Menikoff, Jerry, and Edward P. Richards. 2006. *What the Doctor Didn't Say*. New York: Oxford University Press.

Metcalfe, Rebecca K. and Jay J. H. Park. 2024. "Diversity action plans in clinical trials." *Journal of the American Medical Association*. Published online September 20. Accessed September 24, 2024. doi:10.1001/jama.2024.16009.

Mehta, Neil K., and Virginia W. Chang. 2009. "Mortality attributable to obesity among middle-aged adults in the United States." *Demography* 46(4) (November): 851–872.

Miller, Franklin G., and Howard Brody. 2003. "A critique of clinical equipoise: Therapeutic misconception in the ethics of clinical trials." *Hastings Center Report* 33(3) (May–June): 19–28.

Miller, Franklin G., and Howard Brody. 2007. "Clinical equipoise and the incoherence of research ethics." *Journal of Medicine and Philosophy* 32(2) (March–April): 151–165.

Minnesota Department of Public Health. Swim Lane Map. 2023. Accessed June 26, 2023. https://www.health.state.mn.us/communities/practice/resources/phqitoolbox/swimlanemap.html.

National Cancer Institute NCI Clinical and Translational Research Operations Committee. 2014. "Policy of the National Cancer Institute for data and safety monitoring of clinical trials." Accessed April 21, 2024. https://deainfo.nci.nih.gov/grants policies/datasafety.pdf.

National Commission for the Protection of Human Subjects of Biomedical and Behavioral Research. 1979. *The Belmont Report: Ethical Principles and Guidelines for the Protection of Human Subjects of Research*. Bethesda, MD.

National Eye Institute. 2021. "Guidelines for data and safety monitoring of clinical trials." Accessed April 21, 2024. https://www.nei.nih.gov/grants-and-training/policies-and-procedures/guidelines-data-and-safety-monitoring-clinical-trials.

National Institutes of Health. 1998. "NIH Policy for Data and Safety Monitoring." Accessed April 21, 2024. https://grants.nih.gov/grants/guide/notice-files/not93-084.html.

Obasogie, Osagie K. 2014. "Back to the future: Examining the Institute of Medicine's recommendations to loosen restrictions on using prisoners as human subjects." In *Human Subjects Research Regulation: Perspectives on the Future*, edited by I. Glenn Cohen and Holly Fernandez Lynch, 93–106. Cambridge, MA: MIT University Press.

Omenn, Gilbert S., Gary E. Goodman, Mark D. Thornquist, John Balmes, Mark R. Cullen, Andrew Glass, James P. Keogh, et al. 1996. "Effects of a combination of beta carotene and vitamin a on lung cancer and cardiovascular disease." *New England Journal of Medicine* 334(18) (May 2): 1150–1155.

Parasidis, Efthimios. 2014. "Classifying military personnel as a vulnerable population." In *Human Subjects Research Regulation: Perspectives on the Future*, edited by I. Glenn Cohen and Holly Fernandez Lynch, 65–78. Cambridge, MA: MIT Press.

Persad, Govind. 2014. "Democratic deliberation and the ethical review of human subjects research." In *Human Subjects Research Regulation: Perspectives on the Future*, edited by I. Glenn Cohen and Holly Fernandez Lynch, 158–171. Cambridge, MA: MIT University Press.

Petrarca, Robert, Pravin U. Dugel, Michael Bennett, Adiel Barak, Dov Weinberger, Jeffrey Nau, and Timothy L. Jackson. 2014. "Macular epiretinal brachytherapy in treated age-related macular degeneration (MERITAGE): Month 24 safety and efficacy results." *Retina* 34(5) (May): 874–879.

Phelan, Sean M., Diane J. Burgess, Mark W. Yeazel, Wendy L. Hellerstedt, Joan M. Griffin, and Michelle van Ryn. 2015. "Impact of weight bias and stigma on quality of care and outcomes for patients with obesity." *Obesity Review* 16(4) (April): 319–326.

Porter, Joan P., and Greg Koski. 2008. "Regulations for the protection of humans in research in the United States." In *The Oxford Textbook of Clinical Research Ethics*, edited by Ezekiel J. Emanuel, Christine Grady, Robert A. Crouch, Reidar K. Lie, Franklin G. Miller, and David Wendler, 156–167. New York: Oxford University Press.

Proschan, Michael A., K. K. Gordon Lan, and Janet Turk Wittes. 2008. *Statistical Monitoring of Clinical Trials: A Unified Approach*. New York: Springer.

Resnik, David B. 1998. *The Ethics of Science, An Introduction*. New York: Routledge.

Resnik, David B. 2009. "Re-consenting human subjects: Ethical, legal, and practical issues." *Journal of Medical Ethics* 35(11) (November): 656–657.

Rhodes, Rosamond. 2014. "De minimis risk: A suggestion for a new category of research risk." In *Human Subjects Research Regulation: Perspectives on the Future*, edited by I Glenn Cohen and Holly Fernandez Lynch, 32–44. Cambridge, MA: MIT University Press.

Rid, Annette, Ezekiel J. Emanuel, and David Wendler. 2010. "Evaluating the risks of clinical research." *Journal of the American Medical Association* 304(13) (October 6): 1472–1479.

Rivera, Samantha Cruz, Olalekan Lee Aiyegbusi, Jonathan Ives, Heather Draper, Rebecca Mercieca-Bebber, Carolyn Ells, Amanda Hunn, et al. 2022. "Ethical considerations for the inclusion of patient-reported outcomes in clinical research: The PRO Guidelines." *Journal of the American Medical Association* 327(19) (May 17): 1910–1919.

Riviello, Elisabeth D., Tenzin Dechen, Ashley L. O'Donoghue, Michael N. Cocchi, Margaret M. Hayes, Rose L. Molina, Nicole H. Moraco, et al. 2022. "Assessment of a crisis standards of care scoring system for resource prioritization and estimated excess mortality by race, ethnicity, and socially vulnerable area during a regional surge in COVID-19." *JAMA Network Open* 5(3): e221744. Accessed March 21, 2022. https://doi.org/10.1001/jamanetworkopen.2022.1744.

Rosenblatt, Rand. 1978. "Health care reform and administrative law: A structural approach." *Yale Law Journal* 88(2) (December): 243–336.

Ross, Joseph S., Kevin P. Hill, David S. Egilman, and Harlan M. Krumholz. 2008. "Guest authorship and ghostwriting in publications related to Rofecoxib: A case study of industry documents from Rofecoxib litigation." *Journal of the American Medical Association* 299(15) (April 16): 1800–1812.

Sachs, Benjamin. 2010. "The case for evidence-based rulemaking in human subjects research." *American Journal of Bioethics* 10(6) (June): 3–13.

Scanlon, Thomas M. 1998. *What We Owe to Each Other*. Cambridge, MA: Harvard University Press.

Schaefer, Owen G., Ezekiel Emanuel, and Alan Wertheimer. 2009. "The obligation to participate in biomedical research." *Journal of the American Medical Association* 302(1) (July 1): 67–72.

Shah, Seema, Amy Whittle, Benjamin Wilfond, Gary Gensler, and David Wendler. 2004. "How do Institutional Review Boards apply the federal risk and benefit standards for pediatric research?" *Journal of the American Medical Association* 291(4) (January 28): 476–482.

Silverman, Henry J., and Didier Dreyfuss. 2014. "Were there additional foreseeable risks in the SUPPORT Study? Lessons not learned from the ARDSnet clinical trials." *Hastings Center Report* 44(1) (January–February): 21–29.

Silverman, Henry, Sara Chandros Hull, and Jeremy Sugarman. 2001. "Variability among Institutional Review Boards' decisions within the context of a multi-center trial." *Critical Care Medicine* 29(2) (February): 235–241.

Silverman, William A. 1994. "Patient preferences and randomized trials." *Lancet* 344(8928) (October 8): 1023.

Sobal, Jeffery, and Albert J. Stunkard. 1989. "Socioeconomic status and obesity: A review of the literature." *Psychological Bulletin* 105(2) (March): 260–275.

Specker Sullivan, Laura. 2020. "Trust, risk, and race in American medicine." *Hastings Center Report* 50(1) (January): 18–26.

Stair, Thomas O., Caitlin R. Reed, Michael S. Radeos, Greg Koski, and Carlos A. Camargo. 2001. "Variation in Institutional Review Board responses to a standard protocol for a multicenter clinical trial." *Academic Emergency Medicine* 8(6) (June): 636–641.

Stark, Laura. 2012. *Behind Closed Doors: IRBs and the Making of Ethical Research*. Chicago: University of Chicago Press.

Stark, Laura. 2014. "IRBs and the problem of local precedents." In *Human Subjects Research Regulation: Perspectives on the Future*, edited by I. Glenn Cohen and Holly Fernandez Lynch, 173–186. Cambridge, MA: MIT University Press.

SteelFisher, Gillian K., Mary G. Findling, Sara N. Bleich, Logan S. Casey, Robert J. Blendon, John M. Benson, Justin M. Sayde, and Carolyn Miller. 2019. "Gender discrimination in the United States: Experiences of women." *Health Services Research* 54(Supplement 2) (December): 1442–1453.

Swekoski, Don, and Deborah Barnbaum. 2013. "The gambler's fallacy, the therapeutic misconception, and unrealistic optimism." *IRB: Ethics & Human Research* 35(2) (March–April): 1–6.

Thurrell, Matthew J. 2019. "Idiopathic intracranial hypertension." *Continuum* 25(5) (October): 1289–1309.

Truog, Robert D., Walter Robinson, Adrienne Randolph, and Alan Morris. 1999. "Is informed consent always necessary for randomized, controlled trials?" *New England Journal of Medicine* 340(10) (March 11): 804–806.

Urban Institute. 2022. "Obesity across America: Geographic variation in disease prevalence and treatment options." Accessed April 23, 2024. https://www.urban.org /sites/default/files/2022-02/obesity-across-america.pdf.

U.S. Department of Health and Human Services, Food and Drug Administration. 2006. "Guidance for clinical trial sponsors: Establishment and operation of clinical trial data monitoring committees." Accessed April 23, 2024. https://www.fda .gov/regulatory-information/search-fda-guidance-documents/establishment-and -operation-clinical-trial-data-monitoring-committees.

Veatch, Robert M. 2007. "The irrelevance of equipoise." *Journal of Medicine and Philosophy* 32(2) (March–April): 167–183.

Veatch, Robert M. 2009. *Patient, Heal Thyself: How the New Medicine Puts the Patient in Charge*. New York: Oxford University Press.

Viele, Kert, Anna McGlothlin, and Kristine Broglio. 2016. "Interpretation of clinical trials that stopped early." *Journal of the American Medical Association* 315(15) (April 19): 1646–1647.

Villarosa, Linda. 2022. *Under the Skin: The Hidden Toll of Racism on American Lives and the Health of Our Nation*. New York: Doubleday.

Wakim, Paul G., and Pamela A. Shaw. 2018. "Data and safety monitoring." In *Principles and Practice of Clinical Research*, 4th ed., edited by John I. Gallin, Fredrick P. Ognibene, and Laura Lee Johnson, 127–140. Cambridge, MA: Academic Press.

Wall, Michael. 2017. "Update on idiopathic intercranial hypertension." *Neurological Clinic* 35(1) (February): 45–57.

Weijer, Charles, and Monica Taljaard. 2024. "Ethical challenges associated with pragmatic and cluster RCTs." *New England Journal of Medicine* 391(11) (September 19): 969–971.

Wendler, David. 2011. "How to enroll participants in research ethically." *Journal of the American Medical Association* 305(15) (April 20): 1587–1588.

Wendler, David, and Franklin G. Miller. 2008. "Risk-benefit analysis and the net risks test." In *The Oxford Textbook of Clinical Research Ethics*, edited by Ezekiel J. Emanuel, Christine Grady, Robert A. Crouch, Reidar K. Lie, Franklin G. Miller, and David Wendler, 503–513. New York: Oxford University Press.

Wenner, Danielle M. 2018. "The social value requirement in research: From the transactional to the basic structure model of stakeholder obligations." *Hastings Center Report* 48(6) (November): 25–32.

Wertheimer, Alan. 2014. "Non-completion and informed consent." *Journal of Medical Ethics* 40(2) (February): 127–130.

White, Bruce D., Jane B. Jankowski, and Wayne N. Shelton. 2014. "Structuring a written examination to assess ASBH health care ethics consultation core knowledge competencies." *American Journal of Bioethics* 14(1): 5–17.

Wittes, Janet, Elizabeth Barrett-Connor, Eugene Braunwald, Margaret Chesney, Harvey Jay Cohen, David DeMets, Leo Dunn et al. 2007. "Monitoring the randomized trials of the Women's Health Initiative: The experience of the Data and Safety Monitoring Board." *Clinical Trials* 4(3): 218–234.

World Health Organization on Behalf of the Special Programme for Research and Training in Tropical Diseases. 2005. Operational guidelines for the establishment and functioning of Data Safety Monitoring Boards. Accessed April 23, 2024. https:// apps.who.int/iris/handle/10665/69171.

Index

Basic Bioethics

Arthur Caplan, editor

Books Acquired under the Editorship of Glenn McGee and Arthur Caplan

Peter A. Ubel, *Pricing Life: Why It's Time for Health Care Rationing*

Mark G. Kuczewski and Ronald Polansky, eds., *Bioethics: Ancient Themes in Contemporary Issues*

Suzanne Holland, Karen Lebacqz, and Laurie Zoloth, eds., *The Human Embryonic Stem Cell Debate: Science, Ethics, and Public Policy*

Gita Sen, Asha George, and Piroska Östlin, eds., *Engendering International Health: The Challenge of Equity*

Carolyn McLeod, *Self-Trust and Reproductive Autonomy*

Lenny Moss, *What Genes Can't Do*

Jonathan D. Moreno, ed., *In the Wake of Terror: Medicine and Morality in a Time of Crisis*

Glenn McGee, ed., *Pragmatic Bioethics, 2nd edition*

Timothy F. Murphy, *Case Studies in Biomedical Research Ethics*

Mark A. Rothstein, ed., *Genetics and Life Insurance: Medical Underwriting and Social Policy*

Kenneth A. Richman, *Ethics and the Metaphysics of Medicine: Reflections on Health and Beneficence*

David Lazer, ed., *DNA and the Criminal Justice System: The Technology of Justice*

Harold W. Baillie and Timothy K. Casey, eds., *Is Human Nature Obsolete? Genetics, Bioengineering, and the Future of the Human Condition*

Robert H. Blank and Janna C. Merrick, eds., *End-of-Life Decision Making: A Cross-National Study*

Norman L. Cantor, *Making Medical Decisions for the Profoundly Mentally Disabled*

Margrit Shildrick and Roxanne Mykitiuk, eds., *Ethics of the Body: Post-conventional Challenges*

Alfred I. Tauber, *Patient Autonomy and the Ethics of Responsibility*

David H. Brendel, *Healing Psychiatry: Bridging the Science/Humanism Divide*

Jonathan Baron, *Against Bioethics*

Michael L. Gross, *Bioethics and Armed Conflict: Moral Dilemmas of Medicine and War*

Karen F. Greif and Jon F. Merz, *Current Controversies in the Biological Sciences: Case Studies of Policy Challenges from New Technologies*

Deborah Blizzard, *Looking Within: A Sociocultural Examination of Fetoscopy*

Ronald Cole-Turner, ed., *Design and Destiny: Jewish and Christian Perspectives on Human Germline Modification*

Holly Fernandez Lynch, *Conflicts of Conscience in Health Care: An Institutional Compromise*

Mark A. Bedau and Emily C. Parke, eds., *The Ethics of Protocells: Moral and Social Implications of Creating Life in the Laboratory*

Jonathan D. Moreno and Sam Berger, eds., *Progress in Bioethics: Science, Policy, and Politics*

Eric Racine, *Pragmatic Neuroethics: Improving Understanding and Treatment of the Mind-Brain*

Martha J. Farah, ed., *Neuroethics: An Introduction with Readings*

Jeremy R. Garrett, ed., *The Ethics of Animal Research: Exploring the Controversy*

Books Acquired under the Editorship of Arthur Caplan

Sheila Jasanoff, ed., *Reframing Rights: Bioconstitutionalism in the Genetic Age*

Christine Overall, *Why Have Children? The Ethical Debate*

Yechiel Michael Barilan, *Human Dignity, Human Rights, and Responsibility: The New Language of Global Bioethics and Bio-Law*

Tom Koch, *Thieves of Virtue: When Bioethics Stole Medicine*

Timothy F. Murphy, *Ethics, Sexual Orientation, and Choices about Children*

Daniel Callahan, *In Search of the Good: A Life in Bioethics*

Robert Blank, *Intervention in the Brain: Politics, Policy, and Ethics*

Gregory E. Kaebnick and Thomas H. Murray, eds., *Synthetic Biology and Morality Artificial Life and the Bounds of Nature*

Dominic A. Sisti, Arthur L. Caplan, and Hila Rimon-Greenspan, eds., *Applied Ethics in Mental Healthcare: An Interdisciplinary Reader*

Barbara K. Redman, *Research Misconduct Policy in Biomedicine: Beyond the Bad-Apple Approach*

Russell Blackford, *Humanity Enhanced: Genetic Choice and the Challenge for Liberal Democracies*

Nicholas Agar, *Truly Human Enhancement: A Philosophical Defense of Limits*

Bruno Perreau, *The Politics of Adoption: Gender and the Making of French Citizenship*

Carl Schneider, *The Censor's Hand: The Misregulation of Human-Subject Research*

Lydia S. Dugdale, ed., *Dying in the Twenty-First Century: Towards a New Ethical Framework for the Art of Dying Well*

John D. Lantos and Diane S. Lauderdale, *Preterm Babies, Fetal Patients, and Childbearing Choices*

Harris Wiseman, *The Myth of the Moral Brain*

Arthur L. Caplan and Jason Schwartz, eds., *Vaccine Ethics and Policy: An Introduction with Readings*

Tom Koch, *Ethics in Everyday Places: Mapping Moral Stress, Distress, and Injury*

Nicole Piemonte, *Afflicted: How Vulnerability Can Heal Medical Education and Practice*

Abigail Gosselin, *Mental Patient: Ethics from a Patient's Perspective*

Laurie Zoloth, *May We Make the World?*

Robert Baker, *Making Modern Medical Ethics*

Margaret Battin, *Sex and the Planet: What "Opt In" Reproduction Could Do for the Globe*

John R. Shook and James Giordano, *Bioethics and Brains: A Disciplined and Principled Neuroethics*

Erice Racine, *The Theory of Deliberative Wisdom*

Deborah R. Barnbaum, *Data Safety Monitoring Boards: A Bioethical Perspective*

Publisher contact:
The MIT Press
Massachusetts Institute of Technology
77 Massachusetts Avenue, Cambridge, MA 02139
mitpress.mit.edu

EU Authorised Representative:
Easy Access System Europe, Mustamäe tee 50,
10621 Tallinn, Estonia
gpsr.requests@easproject.com

Printed by Integrated Books International,
United States of America